The Menopause Odyssey

From Hot Flashes to Hormonal Harmony

A Woman's Guide to Thriving Through Menopause and Embracing Aging Gracefully

Valerie Anderson

© **Copyright 2024 - All rights reserved.**

The content contained within this book may not be reproduced, duplicated or transmitted without direct written permission from the author or the publisher.

Under no circumstances will any blame or legal responsibility be held against the publisher, or author, for any damages, reparation, or monetary loss due to the information contained within this book, either directly or indirectly.

Legal Notice:

This book is copyright protected. It is only for personal use. You cannot amend, distribute, sell, use, quote or paraphrase any part, or the content within this book, without the consent of the author or publisher.

Disclaimer Notice:

Please note the information contained within this document is for educational and entertainment purposes only. All effort has been executed to present accurate, up to date, reliable, complete information. No warranties of any kind are declared or implied. Readers acknowledge that the author is not engaged in the rendering of legal, financial, medical or professional advice. The content within this book has been derived from various sources. Please consult a licensed professional before attempting any techniques outlined in this book.

By reading this document, the reader agrees that under no circumstances is the author responsible for any losses, direct or indirect, that are incurred as a result of the use of the information contained within this document, including, but not limited to, errors, omissions, or inaccuracies.

Table of Contents

Introduction 1

Chapter 1
Understanding Your Body Through Menopause 5

The Stages of Menopause 6
Hormonal Changes During Menopause 8
Potential Symptoms of Menopause 10
Getting Diagnosed 11
Risk Factors Associated With Postmenopause 11

Chapter 2
Voices of Menopause—Diverse Stories and Shared Experiences 15

You Are Not Alone 16
    Debbie's Heart Scare 16
    Suzanne's Change in Training 17
    Nicole's Improved Sex Life 18
    Jessica's Chemotherapy and Hormone Replacement Therapy 19
    Jeanine's Menopause and Her Daughter's Puberty 20
Find Your Community 21

Chapter 3
Hormonal Harmony—A Balanced Approach to Hormone Replacement Therapy and Beyond ... 25

What Is Hormone Replacement Therapy? ... 26
Types of Hormone Replacement Therapies ... 27
Benefits of Hormone Replacement Therapy ... 30
Possible Side Effects of Hormone Replacement Therapy ... 30
Potential Risks of Hormone Replacement Therapy ... 31
Exploration of Alternative Treatments ... 33

Chapter 4
Nature's Allies—Exploring Holistic and Natural Remedies ... 35

Manage Your Menopause Naturally ... 36
Stress and Menopause ... 39
Mental Wellness Strategies ... 43

Chapter 5
Nourishing Body and Soul—Tailored Diet and Exercise for Menopause ... 45

Look at Your Diet ... 46
   The Galveston Diet ... 49
Movement for Long-Term Health ... 52
Manage Your Weight ... 53

Chapter 6
Age with Elegance—Positive Aging and Proactive Health Strategies 55

Embrace Aging With a Positive Attitude 56
Develop a Healthy Mindset 57
Tips for Maintaining Vitality and Resilience 58

Chapter 7
Emotional Resilience—Navigating Mood Swings and Mental Health 61

Understand Your Mood Swings 62
Manage Your Emotions 64
Modern Approaches to Mental Wellness 66
Encourage Self-Care 69

Chapter 8
Relationships Reimagined—Fostering Connection and Intimacy 75

Understanding Changes in Intimacy 76
Building Strong Relationships 79
Nurturing Social Support 81

Chapter 9
Staying Informed and Empowered—The Future of Menopause 85

The Evolution of Understanding Menopause 86
The Future of Menopause 87
Menopause From the Male Perspective 88

Chapter 10
Your Menopause, Your Power—A Journey of Transformation 93

Tools for Implementation 97

Perimenopause Symptom Tracker 97
Preparing for Your Doctor's Visit 99
Applications to Consider Using 102

Glossary 105
Acknowledgments: A Note of Gratitude 107
References 109

Introduction

You wake up after yet another restless night. Your pajama shirt is sticking to your skin, drenched from sweat. *It was just a normal Spring night. How is it even possible to be so hot?*, you wonder while you drag your tired body to the shower. You have to pause numerous times while you're washing your hair to remove loose strands that have fallen out and became entangled around your fingers. *At the rate my hair is falling out, I'm going to bald before Christmas*, you think in disgust.

When you're finally on your way to work, you catch a glimpse of yourself in the car's rearview mirror. To your absolute shock, there is even more hair on your chin than the previous time you looked. To make matters even worse, a few of these new hairs are pitch black. You dig in the middle compartment of your car to find a pair of tweezers; these days, carrying tweezers with you is almost as important as taking your phone when you leave the house. While stopped at a traffic light, you're plucking away, constantly keeping an eye on fellow motorists in the hopes that no one you know will see your makeshift beauty treatment in the car. *Oh, this is so embarrassing. Am I actually growing a beard now? Perhaps, I should consider going for laser hair-removal therapy. Why can't these hairs grow on my head where I am losing hair fast? This can't go on like this*, you think.

Throughout your day at the office, you pay almost as much attention to trying your best to keep your pelvic muscles as tight as possible as you do to your actual work. Every time you sneeze, cough, or laugh, you cross your legs, hoping not to leak and end up smelling like an old toilet by the end of the day. *Things just aren't as they used to be*, you think as your panty liner gradually fills due to incontinence. *Maybe I should start wearing full sanitary pads. Since my period has become close to nonexistent, I might as well use the ones still lying in my vanity drawer in the bathroom.*

The rest of the day feels like a blur as you try to navigate other struggles you suddenly have to deal with: Your heart seems to be competing in a marathon, the way it's racing at times; you get pins and needles in your extremities for no apparent reason; your anxiety levels are sky high; and you continuously have to resist the urge to scratch down there. Because not just has your vagina gone drier than a desert, you just can't shake the itch that has become part of your daily life.

If any of this sounds even remotely like your new struggles, you're not alone. Not even close. Menopause affects millions of women worldwide in many different ways. This phase is so much more than just the end of a woman's monthly menstrual cycle. Yes, that is often the most obvious sign of this change of life, as menopause is often referred to, but by the time you realize that your monthly visitor isn't as regular as you're used to, the hormonal changes that accompany this phase are likely in full force already. It is typically the drop in these hormones, particularly estrogen, that causes many of the unpleasant symptoms you're likely struggling with, including those hot flashes that result in you switching on the air conditioner on even the coldest day. In reality, menopause can start months before your period starts to become irregular and is only set to be complete once your period has stopped for an entire year. The transition period that happens before true menopause takes over is called *perimenopause*.

While this is the most natural process all women go through, it affects us all in different ways. For example, vaginal atrophy (dryness and itching) can be unbearable for some women, while others might not be affected by this at all. Also, some women will start showing signs of menopause in their 30s, while others might not experience their first symptoms until they are close to 55. A lucky few might not even have any symptoms and only realize they're menopausal once their monthly visitor has been absent for a while. Menopause has never been a uniform experience. This is why it's so important to understand this change of life so that you'll know you aren't going crazy when you experience symptoms none of your friends or family members might have. You'll even realize that, in making some changes, your symptoms can be completely manageable.

This complete knowledge will serve you well when you have to consider potential treatments for your symptoms of menopause. Many women are hesitant to use hormone replacement therapy out of fear of increased risks of cancer and cardiovascular disease. Some prefer to use natural remedies. However, most of these treatments have evolved drastically over the years, and because everyone has unique health risks and needs, it's always best to create a personalized plan for your health.

What's more, menopause doesn't have to bring about the end of your sex life. While there may be an additional need for lubrication, medication, or even trying out different positions to reduce any pain you might experience, you can enjoy intimacy for many years to come. In fact, you can make many positive changes to your lifestyle that will give you the upper hand over your symptoms and help you thrive. You can regain control over your life and write your own story.

In *The Menopause Odyssey: From Hot Flashes to Hormonal Harmony*, we'll not only unpack all the myths and the latest research that has to do with this change of life but also look at many tips and tricks that can make this phase a lot easier on you and your relationship with your partner. You don't have to go through this stressful and uncertain time alone. This book will be the trusted friend who will not only help you through the ups and downs of menopause but also answer all the questions you might be too shy to ask a friend or even your doctor. You aren't meant to struggle by yourself, no matter what phase of life you're in.

I understand exactly what you're going through and how scary this time can be. My firsthand experience with these turbulent hormonal changes has equipped me with a unique perspective, not just in my professional capacity but also on a deeply personal level. I have helped countless other women understand the many misconceptions that exist around menopause, find remedies suited to their individual needs, and fight the silent battles that too many of us face during this critical stage of life.

The Menopause Odyssey: From Hot Flashes to Hormonal Harmony stands as a testament to a relentless pursuit of holistic solutions, modern insights, and innovative strategies tailored for contemporary women. My approach transcends the conventional, merging tried-and-tested wisdom with cutting-edge research and heartfelt empathy. This book is a call to arms—a declaration that the journey through menopause is not a solitary trek but a shared voyage, rich in challenges, triumphs, and transformative moments.

While many of the symptoms of menopause are unavoidable, you can navigate this by making changes to your lifestyle and choosing a treatment option that works for you. With the correct knowledge and support, you can empower yourself to overcome any challenges this phase of your life may bring and avoid being a victim of your symptoms.

Embrace the odyssey with me and discover the power of updated and insightful solutions. Become part of a community of women who are rewriting the narrative of menopause. Together, let's navigate the waves of change with grace, empowerment, and a renewed sense of vitality.

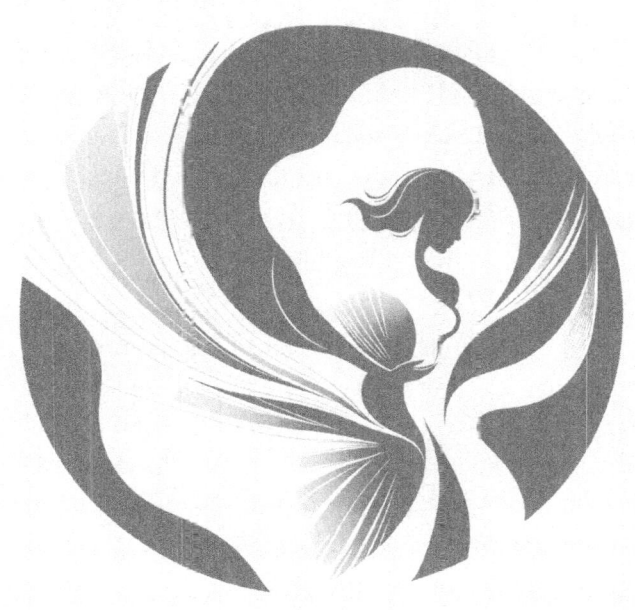

CHAPTER

Understanding Your Body Through Menopause

Can you remember that day when you first got your period? You were likely in your tweens or early teens. Your mother, caregiver, teacher, or guidance counselor at school probably explained this initial change of life all girls experience, so when you first saw blood on the toilet paper after you wiped yourself, you probably understood what was happening to your body. Or perhaps you had no idea what this blood was about, resulting in you freaking out until you got the hang of your cycle and how to use the feminine hygiene and sanitary products that would become part of your life.

In a way, you might have been excited about finally meeting your new monthly visitor, as it was a sure sign that you were entering womanhood. But, on the other hand, this might have been a very scary time for you, as all these changes to your body signaled that your body, as you knew it, would change forever. Fast-forward many years: You're now saying goodbye to this visitor, as menopause is well and truly a new part of your life.

Going through menopause can be a very similar experience to surviving puberty. There are many changes happening to your body that you not only have very little control over but will alter your body for the rest of your life. However, you can learn to deal with the many symptoms that accompany this time and even claim many different victories along the way. But first, let's look at what menopause entails, starting with the different stages of menopause.

The Stages of Menopause

Menopause starts long before your menstrual cycle becomes irregular or disappears, and also goes far deeper than this one obvious sign. Yes, it does signal the end of a woman's fertile years in that she will stop producing eggs on a monthly basis, but with it comes a decline in reproductive hormones, which can last a few months, if not years. For most women, this decline in hormones starts between the ages of 40 and 55. However, it can happen a lot earlier than that; some women start to experience signs of menopause in their early 30s. This is typically the case when they've had their ovaries removed surgically at a young age or when they experience premature ovarian failure.

Menopause can be divided into three different stages, each with its own symptoms that you'll have to learn to manage and triumphs you can achieve by making some changes to your life. Understanding these three stages will not only help you identify the one that you're in but also assist you in choosing the right treatment for yourself:

- **Premenopause or perimenopause:** This is the start of menopause, when your ovaries will start their atrophy, which is basically the degeneration of organ cells. This results in a decline in the reproductive hormones, predominantly estrogen and progesterone, which stimulate the release of an egg and the subsequent menstrual cycle. While women in the perimenopausal stage can still get pregnant, their fertility will gradually decline. If you suspect you're in this phase of life and don't want to have another baby, it's important to continue taking contraceptives until a doctor confirms you're in full menopause. This perimenopausal stage can last for seven years, or even longer, and women often won't realize they're perimenopausal unless they go for a gynecological checkup or have blood tests done. During this time, you may find your periods becoming more irregular; in some months, your cycle will be shorter than the average 28 days, while in other months, it can be significantly longer. You may also experience mood swings and other symptoms of menopause, which we'll discuss below.

- **Menopause:** This stage of life is typically confirmed once your period has been absent for 12 consecutive months. However, before a doctor diagnoses you as menopausal, they will first make sure there aren't any other illnesses, medication, or a possible pregnancy resulting in the absence of your cycle. Once menopause is confirmed, you can no longer get pregnant. On average, this happens around the age of 51, but it can be earlier or later, depending on your individual health and risks.

- **Postmenopause:** This is the stage that follows your fertile years having passed. Your ovaries will still produce low estrogen and progesterone levels, but they will be too low to activate a menstrual cycle. Since your periods will never come back, you'll be classified as postmenopausal for the rest of your life. You might continue to have some of the symptoms you've experienced during perimenopause and menopause, but these will gradually become easier to deal with, especially if you empower yourself in managing them by making certain lifestyle changes. Unfortunately, the lower levels of reproductive hormones can increase your risk of developing conditions such as osteoporosis and heart disease. Luckily, these risks can be mitigated by following a healthy diet, being physically active, and leading a healthy lifestyle. Alternatively, you can consider using hormone-replacement treatments or natural remedies to increase the estrogen in your body. We'll look at all of these options in later chapters.

No matter what stage of this change of life you may find yourself in or how intense your symptoms might be, always remember that there is light at the end of the tunnel. You have the absolute power within you to change your outcome and improve the quality of your life in the process.

Hormonal Changes During Menopause

I've mentioned a few times that hormonal changes, specifically related to your reproductive hormones, take place during menopause. However, unless you have medical training, you may not know how these changes can actually affect your life. Let's take a deeper look at these hormones, their functions, and how their decline during menopause can affect your life (*Changes in Hormone Levels, Sexual Side Effects of Menopause*, 2019):

Hormone	Estrogen	Progesterone	Testosterone
Purpose of this hormone	Promotes and stimulates the growth of breast tissue	Prepares the uterine lining once a fertilized egg attaches to it	Although this hormone is more common and important in the reproductive health of men, it also plays a vital role in a woman's sexual health.
	Maintains the health of the vagina, which includes promoting blood flow to the organ; improves elasticity; and lubricates this external sex organ	Promotes the early health of a pregnancy	Promotes the production of estrogen
	Causes the thickening of the uterine lining during menstrual cycles		Increases libido and sexual desire
	Preserve the health of your bones		Maintains muscle and bone mass

Hormone	Estrogen	Progesterone	Testosterone
The effect of this hormone's decline during menopause	Estrogen levels will change during perimenopause but may do so irregularly. For example, one month your body may produce an excess of estrogen, while the very next, your estrogen levels can be low. As menopause progresses, your estrogen levels will gradually decrease to a very low level.	Your body's production of progesterone stops every month during your monthly cycle if there is no fertilized egg. Once your period stops due to menopause, your body won't produce this hormone anymore.	Testosterone levels in women peak during their 20s. By the time they reach menopause, their levels of testosterone will be around half of what they were during their younger years. After your ovaries' production of estrogen declines, they will continue to produce testosterone. Your adrenal glands will also continue to produce this hormone.
The postmenopausal effects of having low levels of this hormone	The effects of the changes of estrogen levels will depend on how your body's production has changed. While your body produces high levels of estrogen, you might experience heavy bleeding during periods, bloating, and breast tenderness. Once your body produces low levels of estrogen, you might experience many unpleasant symptoms, including hot flashes, palpitations, insomnia, night sweats, vaginal dryness, and bone loss.	The lack of progesterone in your body can result in irregular periods, which can include heavy bleeding and longer cycles.	Your sexual desire may be severely decreased, making it more difficult for you to get into the mood. You may suffer a loss in muscle and bone mass, which can result in you falling and getting injured more often. As the balance of estrogen and testosterone in your body gets altered, with your testosterone levels becoming higher than your estrogen levels, it can result in unwanted hair growth.

Always remember that menopause is not a uniform process, and the decline in these sexual and reproductive hormones can affect women differently. While we'll discuss these changes in more detail in the coming chapters, it's always best to consult your doctor should you ever feel concerned about any symptoms you might experience. You should never feel ashamed to discuss, for example, that funky odor or uncomfortable itch. It can be perfectly normal, and the chances are good that there will be an ointment or other form of treatment that will help you feel a lot more comfortable.

Potential Symptoms of Menopause

Because menopause can present in many different ways, this time can be exceptionally confusing, particularly when you feel unsure whether your change of life has started. This is why it's important to be aware of the many different symptoms to accompany this phase of life. These are the most common symptoms that can start in perimenopause and continue until your period has ended and menopause has been confirmed:

- Hot flashes
- Elevated heart rate
- Vaginal dryness, which can result in pain and discomfort during sex
- Decreased libido
- Urinary incontinence
- Mood changes, which can include irritability, anxiety, and depression
- Night sweats
- Insomnia, sleep disturbances, and fatigue

Many of these symptoms can continue after you've reached the postmenopausal stage of life. However, as we've discussed, most of these will either gradually decrease in intensity or go away completely. These can include:

- Changes in your weight
- Sexual discomfort
- Change in sex drive
- Dry skin
- Insomnia
- Depression

- Night sweats
- Hot flashes
- Hair loss
- Urinary incontinence

The good news is that most, if not all, of these symptoms can easily be managed. However, if your symptoms increase in intensity, even after you've reached postmenopause, it's best to consult your doctor to make sure you don't have any underlying conditions that could contribute to your symptoms.

Getting Diagnosed

If you suspect you might have reached perimenopause, it's best to have this change of life confirmed by a doctor. In most cases, this will be a gynecologist who specializes in female reproductive health. There are, however, some primary healthcare physicians who also treat menopause, so it's best to find out if your general practitioner deals with female health—if you want them to treat your menopause.

If your period has been absent for 12 months and you don't have any underlying conditions that might have caused your missing menstrual cycle, your doctor will likely diagnose postmenopause without doing extensive testing. This is why it will be helpful to track your period once you've noticed that it's becoming irregular—it will help your doctor make a diagnosis. Your doctor may opt to monitor your cycle for a few months before making the official diagnosis.

If you haven't progressed to this final stage yet, your doctor will likely do a variety of tests to diagnose your menopause. Although it may be different in your case, these tests typically include blood tests to check your hormone levels, a pap smear, a pelvic exam, and a breast exam. They may also test your follicle stimulation hormone levels, as these will increase as your ovaries' function starts to decrease. In some cases, they may order a mammogram to check your breast tissue for lumps.

Risk Factors Associated With Postmenopause

While many women are relieved when the severity of their symptoms starts to decrease during postmenopause, this final stage can come with some challenges. Even though the main focus of *The Menopause Odyssey* will be on the journey that leads to this phase, it is important to be aware of the various risk factors that are associated with this time of your life. This will help you plan for what you may experience in your future and know when you need to go to the doctor for a potential further diagnosis and possible treatment.

Some of the risk factors for postmenopausal women include:

- **Cardiovascular disease:** Estrogen plays an important role in protecting women against many different cardiovascular diseases, which include heart disease, heart attack, and stroke. Your lifestyle can play a major role in how negatively your cardiovascular health is affected by the drop in estrogen. For example, if you have a sedentary lifestyle and don't do frequent workouts, your risk for high blood pressure and high cholesterol will be increased, which poses another threat to potential cardiovascular disease. Becoming more active in your lifestyle and eating a healthy diet can go a long way in decreasing the risk that your lower estrogen levels can pose to the health of your heart.

- **Osteoporosis:** As you age, your body naturally loses bone mass. Once your estrogen levels decrease during menopause, your bone density will decrease, as well. This puts you at risk for increased fractures during falls or injuries as well as osteoporosis, a disease that affects the mineral density and mass of your bones. If doctors suspect that you may have low bone health, they can schedule you for bone densitometry, a test that measures the calcium levels in your bones.

- **Vaginal atrophy:** As we've mentioned a few times, menopause can not only result in vaginal dryness, but it can also affect the elasticity of this reproductive organ. Apart from causing sexual discomfort, this atrophy can also impact your entire urinary tract going into your bladder, which can result in urine leaking out of your vagina—known as *incontinence*. Creams and lubricants can help to ease any discomfort your vaginal dryness can cause. If incontinence is a major problem, you can talk to your doctor about options that might be available. This can include laser therapy or even surgery, but it will depend on your individual circumstances.

- **Mental health struggles:** The mood swings that are often associated with menopause can continue well into postmenopause. When you have high levels of depression and anxiety, your stress levels naturally increase. Your vaginal atrophy can also result in challenges in your intimate life, potentially leading to sexual tension with your significant other. If you feel your mental health is suffering as a result of the drop in your hormone levels, and none of your typical strategies at home are working effectively to improve your mood, it will benefit you to speak to your doctor or a therapist to find ways to cope with your challenges more effectively.

Regardless of the stage of menopause you may be in, you should always remember that you're never alone in your struggles. You also don't have to allow your challenges to get the better of you. There are many ways in which you can empower yourself to take back control over your life and your symptoms. In the next chapter, we'll discuss inspirational stories of women who thrived through menopause and found a community among other women.

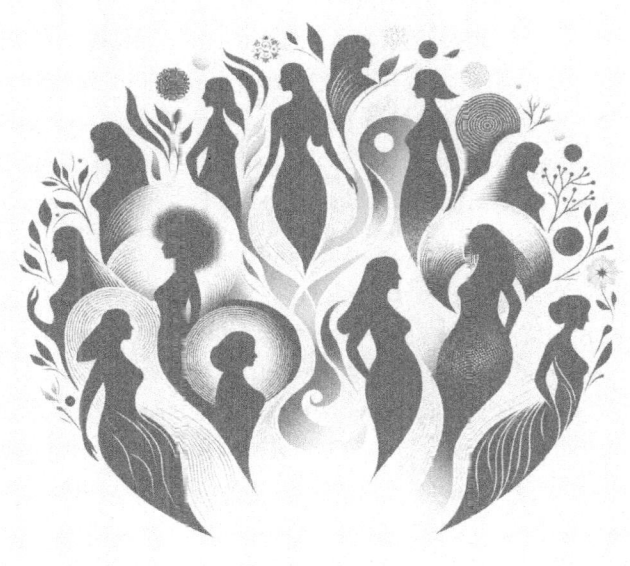

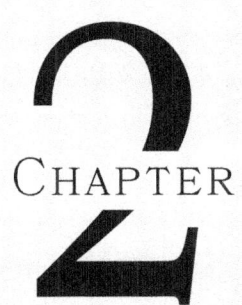

CHAPTER

Voices of Menopause— Diverse Stories and Shared Experiences

Menopause can be an all-consuming stage of life, with new symptoms surprising you continuously. There might be days when you feel like you're living in someone else's body; you might wonder how much of the body you've come to know over the previous decades is still with you. You may also fear that there might be something more seriously wrong with you because your experience of menopause is vastly different from that of your friends or family members.

This is why it can be so helpful to surround yourself with other women going through the same change in life. Being part of a community of other menopausal women will serve as a constant reminder that not only are you not alone in the struggles that can come with this stage of your life, but also will help you realize that the symptoms you experience are absolutely normal. Hearing these women's stories can be both inspirational and empowering, as hearing how other women navigated this phase can help you come up with strategies to make this process more pleasant for you.

You Are Not Alone

Whether you're already part of a community of women in the same stage of life or not, hearing about how others have overcome their struggles can be highly beneficial. To illustrate this, I would like to share a few stories of highly inspirational women I've met on my journey through menopause. While some of their stories and symptoms may seem severe, they were all able to find ways to get past their challenges to find positivity and happiness in the new phase of their lives.

Debbie's Heart Scare

Let's start with the story of Debbie, a 54-year-old woman who had a long and stressful career as the national sales manager of a high-profile company. After her son graduated from college, she decided to give up her job to follow another lifelong dream of hers: owning a coffee shop. She loved this change, and even though running her own business came with challenges, she could happily indulge in a piece of cake when she felt her stress levels getting the better of her.

Things were going great until one morning, when she awoke with a throbbing pain in her jaw. She immediately went to the dentist, who repaired a cavity that was busy forming in one of her left molars. Unfortunately, the pain continued, and she struggled to sleep. A few days later, she was so tired that she decided to close her shop for the day and rest. Unfortunately, before she could get any rest, she experienced the worst pain of her life in her chest, radiating down her left arm. The pain was so intense that she fell to the floor. She had to crawl to her phone to call 911.

Later at the hospital, it was confirmed that not only did Debbie suffer a heart attack, but also that her cardiovascular problems were caused by extremely low levels of estrogen in her body. This confused her as, up to that point, she still got her period fairly regularly. She had no idea that she was already at an advanced stage of perimenopause. The stress of running her own business mixed with her unhealthy lifestyle and cake-eating habits didn't help, either.

While still in the hospital, she consulted with a dietitian about changing her eating habits as well as a psychiatrist about finding healthier coping mechanisms to manage her high levels of stress. She also started a six-week cardiac rehabilitation program, where she was gradually introduced to a workout routine designed for menopausal women. She learned that by making small changes to her life and lifestyle, she could not only rebuild the damage done to her heart but also manage the symptoms of menopause, which soon started in full force, with more ease.

Debbie is now a few years postmenopause and is living her life to the fullest. While she will always have the fear of suffering another heart attack due to her low levels of estrogen, she's doing what she can to improve the health of her heart.

Suzanne's Change in Training

Next, I would like to share the story of Suzanne, a former marathon runner who had to find a new hobby to enjoy. All her life, she enjoyed long-distance running, albeit mostly for fun—although, during her teens and early 20s, she did take part in a few professional marathons. While many other people reach for a cup of coffee after waking up in the mornings, Suzanne reached for her running shoes and would start her days with a quick jog in her neighborhood park.

Unfortunately, when she reached perimenopause, she suffered such severe hot flashes and dizzy spells that running posed too big a risk. During one of her morning runs, she got so dizzy that she almost passed out; had a stranger not helped her to a park bench, she might have seriously injured herself. She had no other choice but to give up running.

Suzanne quickly fell into a deep depression and had to take antidepressants to help her cope with her struggling mental health. During her consultations with a psychiatrist, it became clear that while the hormonal changes due to perimenopause played a big role in Suzanne's diminishing mental health, not being able to go for runs also had a big impact. Her condition got so bad that she didn't want to leave her home. The psychiatrist suggested that Suzanne find other ways of staying active.

Suzanne joined the gym, thinking that doing classes there with other women would be the key to regaining her mental health. One day, while waiting for a yoga class to start, Suzanne kept herself busy on some of the weights at the gym. She enjoyed it so much that she completely forgot about her yoga class. She was, however, still scared that she would injure herself during a dizzy spell—these came without any warning—especially when she was holding heavy weights above her head. To overcome this, she hired a personal trainer to help teach her proper techniques as well as tips to safely put down the weights, should she ever feel dizzy while training. Now, she feels comfortable in her strength and ability and has made a new friend at the gym who has since become her gym buddy.

Six years down the line, Suzanne is in the best health of her life. She has been able to wean herself off the antidepressants, she is physically stronger than ever before, and she has made a good new friend. Menopause empowered her to change her life—for the better.

Nicole's Improved Sex Life

Most women believe that menopause signals the end of their sex life—or, at the very least, the start of a less enjoyable one. If this sounds like your outlook on intimacy during your golden years, Nicole's story might serve as an amazing inspiration and reminder that you can, indeed, have it all.

When Nicole was 18 years old, she went on the pill. She never wanted to have children of her own, so she never had any reason to stop taking contraceptives. When her long-term relationship ended, she decided to go off the pill to give her body a break. Her regular period went away completely, but she didn't think too much about it: Many women struggle with irregular periods when they stop taking contraceptives, so she just assumed that was the cause. Besides, she was only 38 years old, so she believed she was too young for it to be anything else than that.

Six months later, she was in a new relationship and went to the doctor to go back on contraceptives. Her doctor ran routine blood tests before writing the prescription. It was then discovered that Nicole was already postmenopausal. She was extremely confused by this, as the only symptom she ever had was a dryish vagina, something that she wrote off as not being sexually attracted to her previous partner anymore. Since she had no other symptoms, her doctor didn't recommend hormone replacement therapy. She had to find ways to overcome her vaginal atrophy, which largely included using lubrication.

Nicole never felt comfortable discussing sex with anyone, let alone explaining to a new love interest why a woman in her 30s needed lubrication. The conclusion these men always made was that she wasn't attracted to them. That continued for a few years until she eventually met David, a general practitioner. Since he had medical training, he understood her condition and made her feel comfortable enough to talk about sex. For the first time in her life, she could tell her intimate partner what she wanted sexually, which resulted in her enjoying sex again. In fact, she had the best sex of her entire life.

Jessica's Chemotherapy and Hormone Replacement Therapy

Jessica, a mother of two in her 40s, is a breast cancer survivor. After she was diagnosed with breast cancer, her oncologist recommended chemotherapy as treatment. Unfortunately, the aggressive form of chemo she had also brought on menopause, which brought upon symptoms such as brain fog, severe anxiety, weight gain, muscle and joint pain, and extreme fatigue. At first, Jessica believed these symptoms were related to her chemotherapy. However, her doctor indicated that they were actually caused by a drop in her reproductive hormones, a result of her chemo.

She felt completely defeated. Her cancer was in remission, which should be something worth celebrating, but she felt utterly miserable and depressed. Her doctor was hesitant to put her on hormone replacement treatment (HRT) due to the increased risk of breast cancer. She was put on anti-anxiety medication and it was suggested that she change her eating plan to accommodate the symptoms that came with her change in life. Unfortunately, she saw no improvement, which affected her mental health even more. Eventually, her oncologist referred her to a menopause specialist.

After looking through her medical history, the specialist shocked Jessica by suggesting she go on HRT. Her cancer was what specialists referred to as "triple negative," meaning it was not hormone-based. As a result, the increased risk of HRT in cancer is more severe in hormonal cancers. Even though there was still a risk, her current mental state posed a bigger threat to her life. Starting HRT was a risk she was willing to take.

Within a few days of starting HRT, she felt a massive improvement. Her mood lifted almost immediately, and her anxiety levels dropped, as did her brain fog and even the joint pain she experienced. The eating plan she had been following for a while also became a lot more effective, and for the first time in years, she was able to lose weight. Taking the risk on HRT helped Jessica regain control of her life. While there were still days when she was feeling low, these became less frequent.

Jeanine's Menopause and Her Daughter's Puberty

Now, let's look at the story of Jeanine, a woman in her 40s whose reproductive health started declining at around the same time her daughter's started. Yes, at the same time Jeanine went through menopause, her daughter, Mila, started puberty. To say that this was a tough time for this mother-daughter duo would be a massive understatement.

As with many females going through puberty and menopause, this phase of life for mother and daughter started with confusion. Both Jeanine and Mila didn't understand the changes happening to their bodies and why they suddenly had such bad mood swings. They were both constantly irritated, and the smallest things would set them off. Jeanine could feel her relationship with her daughter breaking down and had no idea how to fix it. She never even considered that they were both experiencing changes in life at the same time.

That was until Mila came to her, white in the face, and told her mom that she was bleeding. Jeanine finally realized what was happening to her daughter. As she was getting sanitary products out and showing Mila how to use them, it dawned on

Jeanine that she hadn't had to use these in a while. In fact, when she looked at her calendar, she realized that it had been seven months since she last had a period. She immediately made an appointment with her gynecologist, who confirmed that she was well on her journey through menopause.

After this appointment, she had a frank conversation with her daughter about what they were both going through, why it was affecting them both, and why they fought so often. They agreed that they would both prioritize their self-care, particularly when they felt overwhelmed by the hormonal changes in their bodies. This would include doing deep-breathing techniques, mindful meditation exercises, and focusing on only saying things that would be helpful, not harmful.

While this wasn't a magic cure for their fights, it did help to reduce their arguments and irritation with each other. Also, understanding that the other person's behavior is dictated by the changes in their hormone levels helped both mother and daughter to have more patience with each other. What's more, since they were both going through similar-yet-different stages of their lives, they felt they had something in common.

Find Your Community

Menopause can be a lonely and scary journey if you don't have other people to share in your experience, give your guidance, or simply remind you that you aren't going crazy when the sweat is dripping down your face while everyone around you is putting on another layer. Having others share in your journey will also help you feel like you're part of a community, whether it's simply a group of friends going through the same change in life, or joining an official group for menopausal women.

If you want to join an official community, you should choose one where you'll feel comfortable talking about your experiences. This can be a group in your neighborhood that meets up frequently to discuss all things menopause or even an online community. Think about your life and your personality type and decide which option would work best for you. If you choose to go for an online community, a simple search on the internet or social media will give you a variety of communities to choose from. I would recommend that you join a few of them and remove yourself from communities you don't feel comfortable in until you find the perfect fit for you. If you prefer to have direct contact with people and want to join a community in your area, you can ask your gynecologist, general practitioner, or women's health clinic about groups for menopausal women.

You might even feel like you don't need to join a community and that your group of friends already provides sufficient support during this time of hormonal change. If that sounds like you, I would still encourage you to at least read through the following list of the three most common benefits of being part of a community to make sure you're doing what's right for you:

- **You gain support.** This is perhaps one of the most obvious benefits of being part of a community. When you have the support of other people who understand what you're going through, you'll gain a sense of safety in knowing that you're not alone in your challenges and that what you're experiencing is normal. You'll also gain hope that despite what your situation may look like, you can find ways to overcome your challenges and thrive in life. What's more, you'll get the opportunity to potentially help others by sharing your experiences and telling group members what worked for you.

- **You get a sense of belonging.** Sharing your stories of menopause with other women and being part of that community will help you connect with others and make you feel like you belong. This connection can help you feel valued by people who truly understand what you're going through. When you feel like you belong, you'll be able to cope with negative emotions or experiences more easily.

- **You can gain positive influence.** Hearing the stories of others going through menopause can be extremely inspirational, particularly when they explain how they went about overcoming their challenges. They might give you suggestions you can try in your life, or you can simply draw motivation from the fact that they overcame their challenges and empower yourself to do the same.

While many people might say that you'll gain more benefits the more connections you have, this isn't necessarily true for everyone. Some people, especially those who are introverted by nature and don't like sharing personal stories of their struggles, might benefit most from having only a few trusted people in their community. Always remember that there is no one-size-fits-all approach here. Decide what level and size of community you want in your life and take the necessary steps to create that, if you aren't already part of one.

When I went through menopause, one of my biggest struggles was deciding whether I wanted to use HRT or find natural ways of coping with my symptoms. I was completely conflicted, as what I read on the internet was often contradictory to what my doctor told me. Talking to other women about their views on and experiences with HRT helped me to see the pros and cons of this treatment, which ultimately assisted me in making my decision. In the next chapter we'll take a deeper look at HRT, the benefits of this form of treatment, and the potential risks you should be aware of.

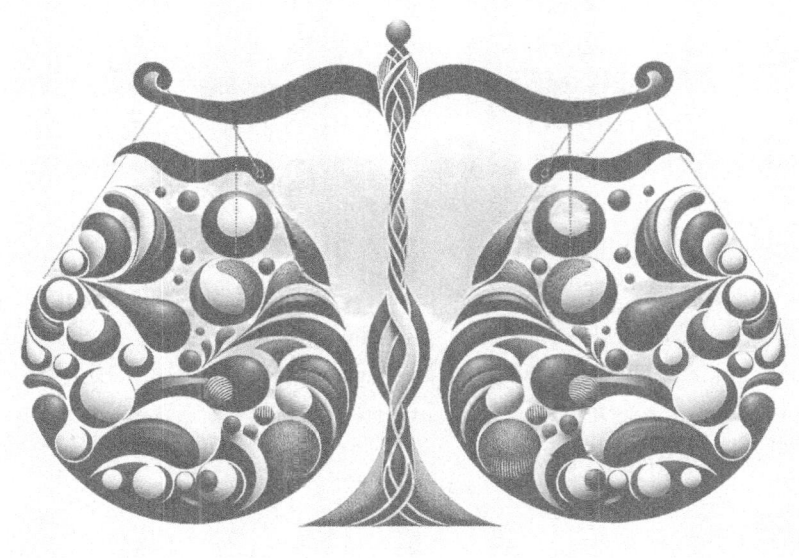

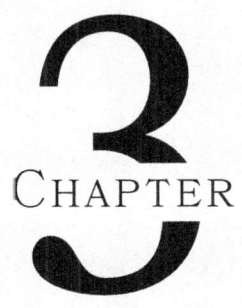

CHAPTER

Hormonal Harmony—A Balanced Approach to Hormone Replacement Therapy and Beyond

Once your doctor confirms that you're on your journey to menopause, whether you're in the perimenopause phase or already in menopause, you need to decide on the treatment that will work best for you. Some people's symptoms are so mild that they can cope with making only slight changes to their lifestyle, while others may need more extensive treatment to minimize the effect of their symptoms in their lives.

One of the most well-known, and perhaps most controversial, treatment options is hormone replacement therapy (HRT). Many women absolutely swear by HRT and believe taking their medication helped them overcome the many challenges that menopause can bring. Others are hesitant to use this form of treatment due to the potential risk factors it could bring to your life.

Always remember that you need to do what is best for you, your body, and your lifestyle. You might have many friends who are against HRT. That doesn't mean you can't or shouldn't choose this treatment. Similarly, if your support system believes HRT is the best way to go, you shouldn't feel forced to also use hormone medicine.

If you educate yourself on HRT and get input from your doctor on what they believe will work best based on your medical history and individual health risks, you can make an informed decision that will help you thrive on your journey through menopause.

What Is Hormone Replacement Therapy?

Before we go into the nitty-gritty of HRT, let's first have a look at what this entails. At the risk of oversimplifying it, HRT involves taking medication to enhance the levels of reproductive hormones—primarily estrogen and progesterone—in women who are experiencing menopause. While some forms of HRT are made bioidentical from plants and other natural matters, others are chemically produced or derived from the urine of pregnant horses. If your doctor believes that HRT will be the best form of treatment for you, they will also recommend the type of HRT that will work best for you.

I recommend that you do your research on the various HRTs before you go to the doctor and jot down any questions you might have. This will help you to ensure you have all the information you may need to make an informed decision on the treatment you choose. Some of the questions you might want to add to your list can include:

- How will HRT benefit me?
- How long will it take before I see and feel improvement?
- What are the potential risks of HRT?
- For how long will I have to take HRT?
- What other form of treatment can I consider?
- Which form of treatment will be best for me?

If you decide on HRT, your doctor will typically start you on a low dose, which might be increased gradually should you need more intense treatment. This will depend on your body's response to the treatment as well as the impact it has on your symptoms. After starting treatment, your doctor will likely schedule a follow-up appointment around three months later to evaluate the effectiveness of the treatment. Once you are both satisfied that you're gaining enough benefits from the treatment, you'll likely only need to see the doctor every six months for a repeat review and prescription.

In most cases, you will end up taking HRT for 2–5 years, depending on the severity of your symptoms. In cases of lengthy menopause or intense postmenopausal symptoms, you might have to remain on this treatment for longer.

Types of Hormone Replacement Therapies

Deciding whether or not you want to use HRT to treat your symptoms of menopause is only one of the many decisions you may have to make. Next, you'll also have to decide on the type of HRT you want to use. There are two main types of HRT to consider (*About Hormone Replacement Therapy (HRT)*, 2023):

- **Estrogen therapy:** This is when medication that only contains estrogen is prescribed and can be in the form of a pill, patch, cream, gel, vaginal ring, or spray. Apart from reducing symptoms of menopause, increasing the estrogen in your body can also help to reduce the impact on your cardiovascular health and the density of your bones. Some of the most popular brand names of estrogen therapy include:
    - **Pills:** Cenestin, Femtrace, Estinyl, Premarin, Estrace, Ogen, and Menest

- **Creams:** Premarin, Estrace, and Ogen
- **Vaginal ring:** Femring and Estring
- **Vaginal tablet:** Imvexxy and Vagifem
- **Patch:** Alora, Menostar, Climara, Vivelle-Dot, Minivelle, Vivelle, and Estraderm
- **Spray:** Evamist

☑ **Estrogen progesterone therapy:** This is also referred to as "combination therapy," as it includes both estrogen and progesterone, or progestin, a synthetic form of progesterone. Some of the most popular brand names of combination therapy include:

- **Pills:** Activella, Bijuva, FemHRT, Angeliq, Premphase, and Prempro
- **Patch:** Climara-Pro and Combipatch

In case you're wondering how you'd decide which type of HRT to use, it's actually rather simple: If you still have your uterus, you'll likely opt for combination therapy. Before you reach menopause, the progesterone in your body assists your body in releasing the endometrium, or the lining of your uterus during, your monthly menstruation. When your body doesn't have sufficient levels of progesterone to release the cells from your endometrium, it can result in an overgrowth of cells in this area, which can become cancerous. By taking additional progesterone, you'll keep this lining thin, which can reduce the risk of uterine cancer.

If your uterus has been removed surgically through a hysterectomy, your body won't have any use for progesterone anymore. As a result, estrogen therapy is recommended.

As you can see above, the different types of HRT come in many different forms, such as gels, pills, and patches. While your doctor will discuss these with you to make a decision, it's good to understand the pros and cons of each of them so that you can be sure to choose one that fits your life and lifestyle (*Hormone Therapy for Menopause: Types, Benefits & Risks*, 2021):

Form of HRT	How it's used	Advantages	Disadvantages
Pills	These are the most common form of HRT and are usually taken once a day.	These pills are generally small and easy to drink.	The risk of blood clots is increased when HRT is taken in tablet form.
Patches	This is another common way of using HRT. The patch is placed on your skin; it gradually releases hormones as your body needs them. The patch typically is replaced every few days, but this depends on the brand of patch you use.	If you struggle to swallow pills or easily forget to take a pill, the patch may be a better option. They don't increase your risk of blood clots, and some of the common side effects of HRT, such as indigestion, can be avoided.	The patches may not stick well on moisturized or sweaty skin. They can also irritate the skin, which can result in itching, and even leave marks on the skin.
Gel	This form of HRT is becoming increasingly popular. The gel is applied to your skin once a day. However, since these gels only contain estrogen, you'll have to add progesterone if you haven't had a hysterectomy.	Similar to the patches, the gel is a good alternative if you struggle to swallow pills or worry about the risk of blood clots.	After you apply the gel to your skin, you need to wait for it to dry and be absorbed into your skin before you can do anything. This can take at least five minutes, so you'll have to add this wait to your timing and planning.
Spray	This spray is used once a day and is applied to either your inner arm or thigh. This spray contains only estrogen, so you'll have to discuss your progesterone needs with your doctor.	The advantages of this spray are similar to patches and gels: They don't contain a risk of blood clots and are an excellent alternative if you struggle to swallow or remember to take pills.	The spray takes approximately two minutes to dry after applying it, so you'll have to give yourself enough time before you get dressed. The wait time to have a shower or bath after applying the spray is an hour, so this will need to be considered in your time-planning.

Form of HRT	How it's used	Advantages	Disadvantages
Vaginal estrogen	This can come in the form of a gel, cream, tablet, or ring. These are inserted into your vagina and can help to reduce the symptoms of vaginal atrophy.	Vaginal estrogen doesn't contain the increased risk of breast cancer that is commonly associated with other forms of HRT.	While vaginal estrogen is effective in treating vaginal atrophy, it won't minimize many other symptoms of menopause, including hot flashes, mood swings, and difficulty sleeping.

Benefits of Hormone Replacement Therapy

While we've already touched on some of the benefits of HRT above, let's look at some of the reasons you might consider using this form of treatment. In short, it helps to minimize the impact that your symptoms of menopause have on your body and life. The most common benefits include reducing hot flashes, vaginal atrophy, night sweats, and itchy skin. Other advantages of taking HRT can include:

- Improved bone health and reduced risk of developing osteoporosis
- Improved mental wellness, including fewer mood swings
- Reduced risk of diabetes, including more control over weight
- Decreased risk of tooth decay and loss
- Reduced risk of many cancers, including colon cancer
- Fewer joint and muscle pains
- Maintained muscle strength

Possible Side Effects of Hormone Replacement Therapy

As with any other medication you may take, HRT can come with some side effects that you'll have to manage. The side effects you can expect can depend on the type of HRT you take (*Hormone Therapy for Menopause: Types, Benefits & Risks*, 2021):

- [x] Estrogen side effects:
  - headaches
  - mood changes
  - diarrhea
  - nausea
  - vaginal bleeding
  - rash or itching
  - leg cramps
  - breast pain and tenderness
  - hair loss
- [x] Progesterone side effects:
  - changes in periods
  - acne
  - headaches
  - mood changes
  - dizziness
  - tiredness
  - nausea
  - diarrhea
  - rash or itchiness
  - breast pain and tenderness
- [x] Side effects of combined type of HRT:
  - headache
  - mood changes
  - vaginal bleeding
  - breast tenderness
  - cramps
  - nausea
  - hives

In most cases, the side effects of taking HRT are so mild that they don't require any intervention. You should be able to continue with your treatment. However, if your side effects are severe or impact your life in a negative way, it's best to discuss this with your doctor. They might change your dosage or even suggest you switch to a different form of treatment that might have fewer side effects. Never change your medication or stop taking it without first discussing it with your doctor.

Potential Risks of Hormone Replacement Therapy

HRT provides the ideal treatment solution for many women who struggle with severe symptoms during menopause. Unfortunately, these treatments don't come without risk. It's important that you consider these potential risks and discuss them with your doctor before you decide whether or not you want to use HRT. Some of the more common health risks include:

- [x] Increased risk of endometrial cancer if you don't include progesterone in your treatment if you still have a uterus

- Increased risk of breast cancer, particularly if HRT is used for an extended time
- Bigger chance of having problems with your gallbladder
- Increased risk of blood clots and stroke
- Bigger chance of dementia if HRT is started too late

There are many things you can do to minimize the potential risks this treatment holds for you. While your doctor will consider this in suggesting a treatment plan, you should be aware of the steps you can take to ensure you're as safe as possible. These can include:

- Start taking HRT within 10 years of the onset of menopause or before you're 60 years old.
- If you still have a uterus, make sure progesterone is included in your treatment.
- Consider other forms of HRT to reduce your risk of blood clots. These can include topical creams, gels, patches, vaginal suppositories, or vaginal rings.
- Go for a pelvic exam and mammogram at least once a year, unless otherwise recommended by your doctor.
- Take the lowest dose of HRT and use it for the shortest possible timeframe.

There may be times when HRT is not recommended and may carry increased risk. Your doctor will consider this, but it's best to also be aware of the factors that may make HRT dangerous, which can include:

- You have abnormal vaginal bleeding.
- You have a history of cancer in the breasts, ovaries, or endometrium.
- You gave had blood clots or risk factors for clotting.
- You have liver disease.
- You have high blood pressure that's either not treated or controlled properly.
- You have a history of heart attack, stroke, or other cardiovascular diseases.
- You suspect that you might be pregnant.

You might think that getting pregnant again is out of the question by the time you start to consider HRT for menopause. However, until menopause has been confirmed, you can still get pregnant if you don't take the necessary precautions. Most doctors will recommend that you continue to use contraceptives even after your period stops. You should use these contraceptives for about 2 years if you're under the age of 50, and at least for a year if you're older than 50. Talk to your doctor about the contraceptive you would like to continue using to make sure it's compatible with the HRT you plan to use.

Exploration of Alternative Treatments

It may be that HRT isn't for you, either due to one of the factors listed above, or you may simply not want to risk the potential dangers that can come with HRT. There are many alternative treatment options that you can consider. No woman should ever feel forced to follow a specific treatment plan. Instead, you should create a personalized treatment approach based on your needs.

In the following chapters, we'll discuss many natural remedies and lifestyle changes that can make it easier to cope with your menopause symptoms. You can also consider trying other types of medicine that can help you thrive on your journey. For example, if you're struggling with severe mood swings, particularly if you have many negative emotions or anxiety, antidepressants can help you reduce mood swings and boost your overall mood. You should, however, consider any potential side effects of antidepressants, which may include feeling shaky, dizzy, nausea, or a reduced libido.

You might also consider taking Clonidine, which is a prescription medication that can help reduce night sweats and hot flashes. Since this medication doesn't alter hormone levels, it doesn't increase your risk of cancer in your breasts or other reproductive organs. Unfortunately, side effects of this medication can include depression, constipation, drowsiness, and a severe dry mouth.

If you're against taking medication or first want to try alternatives before you reach for prescription drugs, there are many natural remedies to consider. In the next chapter, we'll discuss some of these remedies that have been well-tried and tested for helping menopausal women cope with their symptoms.

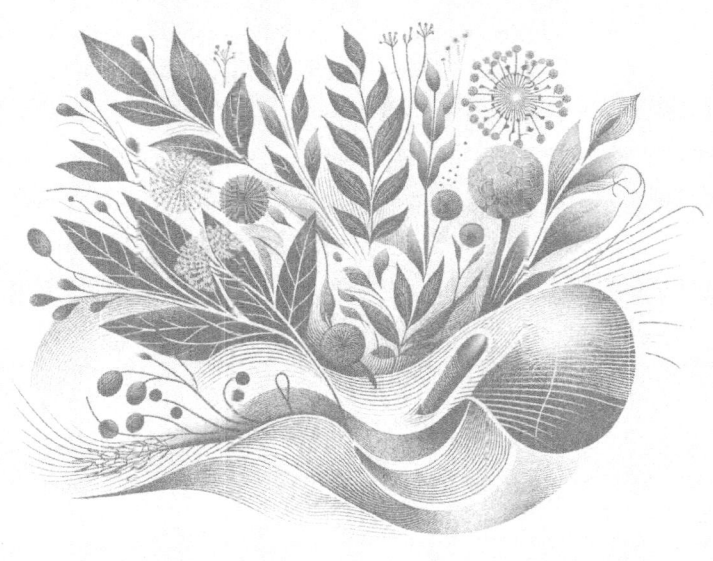

CHAPTER 4

Nature's Allies—Exploring Holistic and Natural Remedies

Many people regard Mother Nature as one of the greatest healers of all time. Spending a few minutes in nature can do wonders to lift the mood and reduce stress and a simple herb can heal many illnesses. It is, therefore, no surprise that many different herbal remedies have been created and developed to treat the symptoms of menopause.

This can provide an ideal alternative for women who either don't want to use medication to help them cope with their symptoms or who have other conditions that can make the use of these unsafe. However, when it comes to these natural remedies, it's important that you do keep in mind that they haven't been tested by the Food and Drug Administration (FDA) as medicine is. Similarly, the manufacturers of herbal medicine aren't required to list all the ingredients or potential side effects. So, even though you may believe that since they are "natural" products, there may still be some risk involved when you take them.

I would always advise that you discuss any herbal supplements with your doctor before you take them—not only to make sure they are truly safe but also that they won't react negatively with any other medication you might take.

Manage Your Menopause Naturally

Let's look at the herbal supplements that are most commonly used to treat the symptoms of menopause, the symptoms they might relieve, as well as the potential side effects associated with them (Ames, 2022):

Herbal remedy	What it treats	Potential side effects
Black cohosh	Reduces hot flashes, night sweats, sleep difficulties, irritability, and vaginal dryness.	Possible gastrointestinal problems, rash, liver damage, and interaction with many prescription medications.
Red clover	Contains phytoestrogens, which are natural alternatives to the hormone estrogen.	Evidence of its benefits for treating symptoms of menopause is inconclusive.

Herbal remedy	What it treats	Potential side effects
Chaste tree berries	Typically used to treat premenstrual syndrome (PMS) and can be effective in treating similar symptoms of menopause.	Nausea, gastrointestinal problems, itching, and headaches. Generally not safe for people with cancer or hormone-sensitive conditions.
Dong quai	Treats menstrual irregularity, period pains, and hot flashes.	Not recommended for women with breast cancer or who take anticoagulants (blood-thinning medications).
Evening primrose oil	Improves hot flashes and PMS breast pain.	Can cause gastrointestinal problems, diarrhea, nausea, and headaches.
Ginseng	Reduces stress, physical exhaustion, fatigue, lack of concentration, hot flashes, and sexual dysfunction.	Can cause postmenopausal vaginal bleeding and shouldn't be used in combination with anticoagulants or medications for high blood pressure.
Hops	Treats hot flashes, anxiety, stress, insomnia, and sexual dysfunction.	Contains phytoestrogen, so shouldn't be used by women with breast cancer or hormone-sensitive conditions. Can react adversely if used in combination with antidepressants.
Horny goat weed	Enhances libido and sexual dysfunction.	Shouldn't be used by people with increased heart rates or palpitations.
Lemon balm	Improves digestion, memory, insomnia, anxiety, and mood swings.	Can cause nausea, dizziness, sedation, wheezing, increased appetite and skin irritation.
Linseed (flaxseed)	Reduces vaginal dryness and inflammation, and improves digestion and menstrual irregularity.	Can cause bloating and increased bowel movements.

Herbal remedy	What it treats	Potential side effects
Maca	Improves sexual function, energy, and mood swings.	Women with cancer and hormone-sensitive conditions should be careful using this supplement. Can make you feel jittery.
Passionflower	Improves mood swings, palpitations, muscular pain, hot flashes, fatigue, and headaches.	Can cause confusion, uncoordinated movements, and drowsiness.
Shatavari	Improves libido, sexual function, and general well-being.	Can cause itchy eyes and skin, skin rashes, dizziness, palpitations, and symptoms of asthma.
St John's wort	Helps treat symptoms of anxiety, insomnia, hot flashes, and irritability.	Shouldn't be used in conjunction with anticoagulants, HIV medication, anticonvulsants, antidepressants, and immune-suppressant drugs.
Tribulus	Improves energy and sexual function.	Can result in stomach aches, diarrhea, and nausea.
Valerian	Improves sleeplessness.	Can cause headaches, diarrhea, palpitations, drowsiness, vivid dreams, and dry mouth.
Wild yam	Improves abdominal and ovarian pain.	Can result in upset stomachs, vomiting, and headaches.
Licorice	Relieves hot flashes and improves sexual function.	Can increase blood pressure and lower the potassium in your body.
Anise	Reduces hot flashes.	Generally believed to be safe to use.
Fennel	Reduces anxiety and depression and improves vaginal atrophy.	Can cause difficulty breathing, chest pain, vomiting, hives, and skin rashes.

Herbal remedy	What it treats	Potential side effects
Pollen extract	Reduces hot flashes.	Can result in dizziness, breathing problems, sores in the mouth, and stomach aches.

Over the years, I've worked with many women with varying opinions on natural remedies and their treatment of menopause. There were some who didn't even want to give them a try, while others absolutely swear by them. One of these women, Maria, had a whole kitchen cupboard filled with different herbs, with the benefits and uses of each of them printed and pasted on the inside of the cupboard door. Whenever she experienced a symptom of menopause, she would look at which herb could help ease her discomfort, and then take it. To make her belief in these herbal medicines even more interesting is the fact that throughout her life, she was a firm supporter of Western medicine and actually laughed when people suggested using herbs... Until her hot flashes got so bad that she reached for evening primrose oil out of desperation. She explained that she felt relief within minutes, something that her HRT couldn't do.

Always keep an open mind and decide what is best for you. If you want to give these natural remedies a try, I would absolutely encourage you to discuss this with your doctor or herbal healer to help you find herbs that could work for you. However, if you don't believe in the power of herbal medicine or if they aren't effective for you, go with what you feel is best for your body and life.

Stress and Menopause

When you're constantly on edge, it can make even the mildest situation seem unbearable. This includes the symptoms of menopause. Unfortunately, regardless of the phase of menopause you might be in, your fluctuating hormones can cause higher levels of stress, which can result in even more mood swings, loss of confidence, feelings of overwhelm, and increased anxiety. I remember how easily I got overwhelmed when I started my journey through menopause and how I suddenly struggled to manage my stress. The more I stressed, the worse my symptoms felt. My hot flashes felt unbearable, my night sweats got so bad that I had to change my bedding almost daily, and controlling my weight seemed to be even more impossible than ever before.

If you're wondering how this works, it all comes down to your stress hormones, cortisol and adrenaline. These are also known as your fight-or-flight hormones. When you experience stress, your body releases these hormones to help you respond as quickly and effectively as possible. Your adrenaline boosts your energy and heart rate, while cortisol increases your blood sugar levels. This enables you to act quickly to protect yourself from the potential threat causing your stress.

Once the potential threat passes, your acute stress and accompanying hormones will go away. However, when you experience chronic or long-term stress, these hormones will remain in your body, which can severely affect many of the natural processes in your body. This includes menopause and its typical symptoms, such as brain fog, mood swings, hot flashes, depression, and exhaustion, all of which can appear to be more pronounced. What's more, increased levels of cortisol for extended periods can also affect the body's production of estrogen and progesterone. By the time you reach perimenopause, your adrenal glands are responsible for producing these reproductive hormones. When they are constantly busy making cortisol, these glands may not make sufficient amounts of estrogen and progesterone, which can fast-track your menopause.

While your doctor can prescribe you medication to help you cope with your stress more effectively, you can also introduce many self-care strategies to help calm yourself, even when your stress levels are through the roof. Some of the strategies that have been very effective for me and countless other women include:

- ☑ **Break your bad habits.** If you have any bad habits that aren't improving your life in any way or might be contributing to your stress, it's best you try to break these as soon as possible. This can include drinking too much, smoking, comfort eating, or overindulging on processed foods or treats with high sugar content. In the next chapter, we'll go into more detail on how you can adjust your diet to help bring balance to your life.

- ☑ **Stay hydrated.** Always remember to drink enough water, as this will not only help you stay healthy but can also lift your mood. Also, if you have a lot of hot flashes and night sweats, your body may need more hydration. You should aim to drink around eight glasses of fluids (water or noncaffeinated drinks) every day.

- ☑ **Move around.** If you have a sedentary lifestyle, your symptoms of menopause may feel worse than if you are active. Unfortunately, if you're constantly feeling hot and lack energy, you may struggle to muster the willpower to do exercises. In the next chapter, we'll discuss various ways you can easily incorporate a workout routine into your life.

- ☑ **Find time to relax.** Apart from incorporating workouts into your life, you should also make time to do things that you enjoy. Whether this is reading, listening to music, doing arts, or even gardening, use this time to unwind and remember all the things you have in your life to be grateful for.

- ☑ **Jot down positive affirmations.** It's natural for everyone to have negative thoughts at times. You need to remind yourself often that these negative thoughts aren't necessarily based on the truth. That's why it's not only important to question whether these thoughts are based on any facts, but also to use positive affirmations to boost your mood. I created a habit of writing down all the positive affirmations that speak to me, and whenever I felt low or had unhelpful thoughts bringing me down, I would read over them until I felt better. I still do this.

- ☑ **Talk about your challenges.** Keeping your frustrations bottled up can become seriously overwhelming. If you can find a release by talking about what's bothering you, you'll not only put yourself in a position to bounce ideas off others but also get advice you might not have thought about yourself. Talking about your problems might even help you to realize that they aren't as bad as you thought they were.

- ☑ **Take deep breaths.** Deep-breathing exercises can be extremely valuable in helping you to calm down and feel relaxed. This is also a simple technique that you can incorporate into your life in any situation you might find yourself in when your symptoms of either menopause or stress get the better of you. While there are many different breathing exercises you can do—a simple online search will teach you how to do them—I prefer doing box breathing. Here are the four simple steps to follow:
  - ◉ Inhale slowly through your nose for five counts.
  - ◉ Hold your breath for five counts.

- Exhale through your mouth (ideally with pursed lips) for five counts.
- Hold your breath for five counts. Repeat this exercise as many times as you need to until you feel calm.

☑ **Visualize positive scenarios.** It often happens that we are so overwhelmed by our challenges, symptoms of menopause, and high levels of stress that we struggle to see a way out. Doing guided imagery can help you visualize pleasant and relaxing environments, which can help you shift your focus from the negatives you might struggle with to the positives you either have in your life or strive to gain. To do this, you can follow these steps:

- Sit or lie in a comfortable position, ideally in a space where you are as free from distractions as possible. I have a comfortable chair in my bedroom that I use to do my meditations and guided imagery; my family knows that when I close my bedroom door, I need a few minutes to myself.
- Think about either a relaxing memory or an environment you feel calm in. If you can't think of one, imagine the perfect scenario. Use all five of your senses to visualize this: what can you see, what can you hear, what can you smell, what can you taste, and what can you touch?
- As you find yourself calming down and your heart rate slowing, focus only on these relaxing sensations.

☑ **Become more mindful.** It often happens that we are so consumed by our stressors or symptoms of menopause that we lose sight of what's really important or happening in our lives. Becoming more mindfulness can help bring the focus back to the present moment, which can help to not only reduce the clutter in our minds but also help you prepare the next step you need to take. Meditating in a mindful manner is very easy to do:

- Sit or lie in a quiet space where you won't be distracted.
- Practice a few rounds of deep breathing until you have settled into a good rhythm.
- Focus only on your breathing. When thoughts pop up in your head or you experience emotions, accept them without judgment and return your focus to your breathing.

☑ **Relax your muscles.** When we are experiencing high levels of stress, our entire bodies are affected by this, often without us realizing it. Doing progressive muscle relaxation will not only help you understand how stress manifests in your body but will also bring calmness and relaxation to your different muscle groups. You can do this exercise alongside mindful meditation, deep breathing, or guided imagery, or as a stand-alone technique. You can follow these easy steps:

- Sit or lie in a comfortable position in an environment relatively free from distractions.
- Settle into a rhythm of deep breathing.
- Start with a specific muscle group—for example, your feet. Contract the muscles for about five seconds, and then slowly release this contraction for about ten seconds. As you do this, focus on how your muscles are feeling and how the tension is leaving your body.
- Continue with the next group of muscles and take it section by section until you've contracted and released all the muscles in your body.

Working on managing and lowering your stress levels can also help to improve your mental health and reduce the impact that any mental illnesses might have on your body and life.

Mental Wellness Strategies

Apart from the increased stress levels affecting your mental health, your fluctuating hormone levels due to menopause can also have an impact on your mental wellness. Many women dismiss this impact, resulting in them facing their battles in silence and not getting treatment that can improve their lives. Some of the most common mental health concerns during menopause can include:

- anxiety
- depression
- low self-esteem
- loss of confidence
- mood swings
- anger
- brain fog and poor concentration

Unfortunately, many of these symptoms start to become more severe during perimenopause. Since a lot of women may not be aware that they are starting this change in life unless they have regular medical checkups, these symptoms may feel completely out of the blue and confusing. I remember how I would jump into a fit of rage, especially at my poor partner, for no obvious reason, or how many times I would waste precious time looking for my phone or the car keys that I was holding my hand. Only once my perimenopause was confirmed did I start to understand that waking up in the middle of the night feeling panicky or placing my grapes in the freezer instead of the fridge weren't signs of me going crazy. It was simply my fluctuating hormone levels affecting me. I started to draw comparisons between how I was feeling during perimenopause and what I could remember from puberty, which also helped me a lot in coping with my mental health struggles.

Apart from the hormonal changes, many women on their journey through menopause experience major changes in their personal lives, as well. Your children might be going through puberty, or even leaving the home, leaving you with empty nest syndrome. You might even have to care for sickly or aging parents, which can add extra pressure on you physically, emotionally, and mentally. However, if you understand the changes in your body and life and know how these changes can affect you in different ways, half the battle in improving your mental health might be won.

It's also important to keep in mind that if you've experienced any form of mental health challenges in the past, which can include postpartum depression, you may be more likely to struggle with these type of issues during perimenopause. You should know the signs of these conditions so that you can take action and seek help when they impact your life. This may include seeking professional help. Medication, therapy, and lifestyle changes can help relieve these conditions. We'll discuss this in more detail in Chapter 7.

Adjusting your diet and making sure you get enough exercise can make a big difference in improving your mental health. In the next chapter, we'll look at lifestyle changes you can make to help you cope with your symptoms of menopause more effectively.

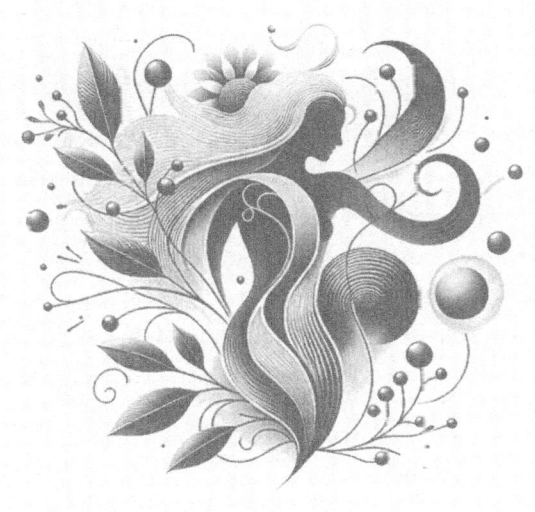

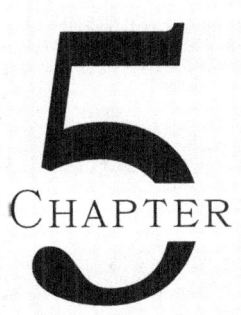

CHAPTER

Nourishing Body and Soul—Tailored Diet and Exercise for Menopause

Whether you choose to treat your symptoms of menopause by taking HRT or natural remedies, making changes to your lifestyle can make a major difference in your life. It can help lessen the severity of your symptoms and even reduce the impact that your decreasing hormone levels can have on your health.

Some of the most obvious aspects you can look at improving are how you take care of your physical body through nutrition and exercise. Doing this the right way, you can even boost your weight loss, which might be something you've been struggling with. I remember how difficult it was for me to lose weight. Throughout my life, I've always taken care of my body and never had any challenges with my weight. However, once I reached menopause, everything changed. Suddenly, I got so much belly fat that I looked pregnant, and none of the diets that had worked for me in the past brought any success.

After doing research, I started to understand why my body wasn't reacting to my typical diets and eating plans the same way as it used to. I realized that I had to make major changes to my nutrition as well as my exercise routine to regain control over my body. I started following the Galveston diet and hired a personal trainer to develop a training program specific for hormonal health. In this chapter, I will share information and tips that have helped me and many other women improve our health.

Look at Your Diet

Let's first look at your nutrition and how you may want to change your diet. When you enter menopause, it's more important than ever to watch what you eat. Not only can the fluctuating hormones result in more weight gain, but the foods that you eat can have a direct impact on the severity of your symptoms. The drop in hormones during menopause can also affect various organs in your body, as well as your cardiovascular health and bone density. These are all aspects you should consider when working out a nutritional plan. While you should have realistic expectations and keep in mind that there will be some symptoms of menopause and aging that you won't be able to change, improving your health by eating properly will help make these symptoms more manageable.

Let's first look at different foods you should include in your diet, as they may help to reduce the severity of many symptoms, including hot flashes, sleeping difficulties, and low bone density (Groves, 2018):

- **Dairy products:** As your estrogen levels decrease, your risk for low bone health and fractures increase. The calcium, potassium, magnesium, phosphorus, and vitamins D and K in dairy products are essential in improving bone health. The amino acid tryptophan found in dairy products can also aid in creating healthy sleep cycles, not only assisting you in falling asleep but also in staying asleep. Apart from dairy products, broccoli and legumes can also boost your calcium.

- **Healthy fats:** While it's important for every person to eat a healthy amount of good fat, women in menopause will also benefit from these fats, which include omega-3 fatty acids. This is particularly important for women who struggle with coronary heart disease or have diabetes. Foods rich in these fats include fatty fish—for example, salmon, tuna, and mackerel—and seeds, such as flaxseed and chia seeds.

- **Whole grains:** These foods are not only rich in B vitamins and fiber but also niacin, riboflavin, thiamine, and pantothenic acids, which are associated with a lowered risk of cancer, heart disease, and premature death. A study conducted in 2021 found that diets filled with whole grains and vegetables can also reduce symptoms of menopause. Examples of whole-grain foods include brown rice, whole-wheat bread, quinoa, oats, rye, and barley.

- **Fruits and vegetables:** Fresh produce is rich in a variety of vitamins, minerals, antioxidants, and fibers; a study found that menopausal women who eat a lot of fresh fruit and vegetables generally have fewer symptoms than those who don't. A study showed that dark berries and strawberries are particularly beneficial, particularly for those struggling with high blood pressure.

- **Phytoestrogen foods:** These are foods that contain high levels of phytoestrogen, which is a natural variant of the reproductive hormone estrogen. As we mentioned in Chapter 4, replacing your hormone levels can provide many menopausal health benefits, including a reduced risk to cardiovascular health and improved bone density. Foods with high levels of phytoestrogen include plums, berries, grapes, peanuts, soybeans, flaxseeds, chickpeas, and barley.

- **Protein:** Including good-quality protein rich in iron in your diet can reduce the impact that menopause can have on the strength of your muscles and bones. For this reason, it's recommended that menopausal women should eat around 0.07 oz of protein per pound of their body weight every day. Taking collagen peptides can also help to boost your bone-mineral density. Foods rich in protein include dairy products, eggs, legumes, meat, and fish. You can also get your iron boost in the form of leafy-green vegetables and nuts.
- **Water:** Always make sure you drink enough water every day. Depending on your lifestyle and level of activeness, it's recommended that you drink around eight glasses of water every day.

While these foods can help to reduce the severity of menopausal symptoms, many other foods can actually make many of these symptoms—particularly weight gain, sleeping difficulties, and hot flashes—even more challenging to deal with. Let's look at some of the foods you should consider limiting in your diet (Johnson, 2022):

- **Trans fats:** These unhealthy fats are often used to make food tastier but carry an increased risk of heart disease and weight gain. Examples of trans fats that you should try to avoid include bacon, margarine, potato chips, sauces, instant soups, breads, cookies, and pastries.
- **Sugar:** Similar to trans fats, sugary treats are high in refined carbohydrates, which can help to give you an instant boost of energy but offer very little sustenance. Instead, these foods can destabilize your blood glucose levels and increase your insulin levels, which can not only wreak havoc with your metabolism but also increase your risk of developing type 2 diabetes.
- **Artificial sweeteners:** Many people opt for artificial sweeteners to compensate for not consuming sugar. These are often found in diet foods and cool drinks, chewing gum, and many candies. Unfortunately, these artificial sweeteners not only affect your body's insulin control but can also negatively impact the balance of the good bacteria in your digestive system.

- **Alcohol:** Although alcohol is generally believed to be detrimental to your health, it's even more important to cut your alcohol consumption when you're on your journey through menopause. Apart from other health concerns, such as damage to your liver, alcohol can also affect your sleep cycles, making it difficult to stay asleep. Alcohol can also increase your core body temperature, which can result in worse hot flashes and night sweats. Another risk that alcohol pose to menopausal women is weight gain. Not only does alcohol contain a lot of calories, but it also stimulates your appetite, which can result in you eating more than you need to.

- **Spicy food:** Hot or spicy food can stimulate many nerve endings in your body, which can cause and worsen hot flashes. It can also upset the balance of good bacteria in your digestive system, which can impact the health of your gut and result in bloating, gas, diarrhea, or constipation. Other foods that can trigger similar reactions can include tomatoes, eggs, and dairy products.

I recommend that, unless you're following a specific diet or eating plan developed for menopausal women, you make a list of the recommended food that you enjoy eating and keep this in mind when you do meal planning or grocery shopping. Alternatively, there are many eating plans you can consider following.

The Galveston Diet

The Galveston diet was life-changing for me in helping me lose my belly fat and improve my overall wellness. This anti-inflammatory eating plan was designed specifically for menopausal women and puts an emphasis on when you eat and what you eat rather than strictly restricting the number of calories you consume. It's largely based on the 16/8 regiment of intermittent fasting, whereby you eat for 8 hours of the day while the other 16 hours form part of your fasting window. This is then combined with a high-fat and low-carbohydrate eating plan of foods with the specific purpose of fighting inflammation in the body.

This diet was originally designed by Dr. Mary Claire Haver, an obstetrician-gynecologist (Nikam, 2021) as she was trying to lose weight while on her journey through menopause. She initially followed the traditional route of restricting her calories and exercising more frequently. However, as many other menopausal women discover, this route wasn't effective anymore.

Haver changed her thinking about weight gain and seriously considered the impact that hormonal changes can have on the amount of weight you carry on your body. She realized that the various food's impact on hormones, as well as the timing of your meals, play a much bigger role in your body's metabolism, especially as you age, than cutting calories. As a result, she developed her Galveston diet based on three components:

- **Intermittent fasting:** As we've mentioned, this diet follows the 16/8 intermittent fasting regime, whereby you're only allowed to eat for 8 hours every day. During your fasting window, you can't consume any calories. Water and unsweetened coffee or tea are allowed. Even though you won't count your calories during your eating window, it generally happens that people eat less. Apart from aiding weight loss, it also helps in reducing inflammation and heart disease as well as improving your body's insulin function.

- **Anti-inflammatory foods:** Inflammation forms part of your body's natural immune response. While short-term inflammation is vital for your body's ability to heal wounds and fight infections, long-term inflammation is linked to an increased risk of cancer, obesity, arthritis, and heart disease, all of which can ultimately have fatal consequences. Foods like vegetables and fruits, which are rich in various plant compounds and highly encouraged in the Galveston diet, have amazing anti-inflammatory qualities.

- **High fat intake:** Where the typical American diet is high in carbohydrates, the Galveston diet emphasizes fats as the major source of nutrition. This provides a fuel refocus, whereby your body uses the fat contents of your food to produce energy instead of relying on carbohydrates.

If you're interested in following this diet, it's best to follow their complete meal plan to ensure you gain the most benefits from this lifestyle change. However, to help you decide whether this is something that may work for you, let's look at the foods this diet encourages you to eat:

Food type	Foods to eat
Fats	Olive oil, coconut oil, avocado oil, butter, and sesame oil
Nuts	Peanuts, pistachios, cashews, and almonds
Proteins	Lean ground beef, lean pork, turkey, chicken, eggs, tuna, trout, salmon, and shellfish
Seeds	Chia, flax, pumpkin, sunflower, and sesame
Fruits	Avocado, raspberries, blueberries, and strawberries
Dairy	Heavy cream, nut milk, sour cream, cheese, and Greek yogurt
Leafy greens	Kale, spinach, dill, lettuce, and mustard greens
Other vegetables	Broccoli, carrots, cauliflower, onion, cabbage, cucumber, bell pepper, and tomato
Fresh herbs	Basil, ginger, thyme, garlic, and parsley
Tea	Chamomile, black, oolong, and green

As with all eating plans, there are many foods that are best avoided when following the Galveston diet:

Food type	Foods to avoid
Sweeteners	Artificial sweeteners and added sugar
Processed foods	Processed meats, refined grains, and fried food
Food additives	Artificial flavors, colors, and preservatives
Vegetable oils	Soybean, corn, sunflower, and safflower
Alcohol	Wine, beer, and spirits
Sugar-sweetened beverages	Soft drinks, juice, and sweet tea

As I've mentioned, there are many eating plans designed specifically for menopausal women. Even though the Galveston diet worked for me, it might be completely different for you. For this reason, I urge you to take your time in finding an eating plan that works for you, your body, and your lifestyle.

Movement for Long-Term Health

Exercise and good nutrition go hand in hand in any healthy lifestyle, regardless of what stage of your life you may find yourself in. Following a proper workout routine can also be valuable in pushing back against many of the symptoms of menopause you might experience, particularly controlling unwanted weight gain and managing soaring stress levels.

Controlling your weight becomes extremely important as you reach midlife. It isn't just about fitting into your favorite pair of jeans from your college years anymore. Now, preserving your health becomes more important. The weight that you gain during midlife often sits around your tummy in the form of visceral fat. This is also the type of fat that poses the biggest risks to your organs, particularly your heart. Also, being more active will help to build strong muscles, which is important as you age and your bones naturally become more brittle. If you have strong muscles protecting your bones, not only will your risk of falling be reduced but also the threat of fractures will decrease.

It's recommended that you aim at doing about 25–30 minutes of exercise 3 times a week. This can be split into 2 sessions a day—for example, 15 minutes in the morning, and another 15 minutes at night. You also don't have to go to the gym to get a good workout. While having access to personal trainers and equipment can make working out easier, there are many exercises you can do in the comfort of your home without spending hundreds of dollars on equipment or a gym membership. There are many exercise videos and applications available online that you can follow free of charge. Alternatively, here are 4 of my personal favorite types of exercises to do:

- **Weight training:** You can buy basic weights for relatively cheap, or there may be many household items you can use as makeshift weights—for example, bottles filled with water can be surprisingly effective as weights. What's more, you can easily do these exercises while watching your favorite show on the TV. Suggestions of exercises you can do while holding weights include punching the air, arm curls, and shoulder overhead lifts.

- **Cardio:** These types of exercises get the heart pumping, which can do wonders in replacing the role that your estrogen used to fulfill in protecting your heart. Doing cardio can also help to elevate your mood and sleep more soundly at night. Examples of cardio exercises you can do include going for a brisk walk, jogging, cycling, and swimming.

- **Yoga:** While you can join a yoga class in your area, you can also easily learn this wonderful form of exercise by following an online video. All you need to do this is a yoga mat. The benefits of yoga are incredible: It helps to reduce your blood pressure, improve your flexibility and mobility, and boost your sleeping cycles. Yoga will also teach you how to relax and calm yourself down, which can do wonders in helping you cope with many of the symptoms of menopause, such as hot flashes and mood swings.

- **Pelvic-floor exercises:** If you struggle with incontinence, doing pelvic exercises can help strengthen your vaginal muscles. Since these exercises boosts the blood flow to your genitals, they can even help to improve sexual arousal and satisfaction during intercourse, which is something many women struggle with as they reach the end of their menopausal journey.

It's never too late to start exercising. Start with something you enjoy and make sure it fits into your schedule. The easier you can include working out and the more fun you can make it, the better the chances will be of continuing with it long-term. Try to include a good mixture of exercises in your routine—cardio or endurance, strength, and balance exercises. Apart from making your symptoms of menopause more manageable, these are also effective in increasing the bone-mineral density of the spine in postmenopausal women.

Manage Your Weight

As we've mentioned, increased weight gain during menopause can cause many health concerns, including breathing difficulties, type 2 diabetes, and cardiovascular disease. While there are no magic ways to prevent or reverse menopausal weight gain, you can manage it by making healthy lifestyle choices, such as:

- Make sure you do regular exercise and eat right, as discussed in this chapter. Also, be more mindful when you eat by focusing on every bite you take. Remove all distractions, such as your phone or the TV, while you eat.

- Look at your sleeping habits and take the necessary steps to ensure you get a good night's sleep. This includes creating the right environment in your bedroom conducive to sleep and reducing screen time for at least an hour before bed. The blue light that devices emit slows down your body's production of melatonin, the hormone that helps you fall asleep.

- Limit your alcohol intake.

- Opt to stand rather than sit as much as you can—for example, install a standing desk to work at if you can and avoid sitting down while you're talking on the phone.

- Park farther away from the store so that you force yourself to walk more. Also, when you go to the bathroom at the office, walk the farthest route instead of taking the shortest, straightest path.

- Spend time in nature to reduce your stress and improve your mental health. If you can, take off your shoes and stand barefoot in the soil, as this will help you connect with nature even more.

Aging is an inevitable part of life. No matter how much you may try to fight it, you can't escape the clutches and challenges that comes with getting older. What you can change, however, is the mindset with which you age. If you have a positive mindset, you'll not only enjoy this journey more, but you'll also be able to deal with any difficulties you may face more effectively. In the next chapter, we'll discuss mindset and how you can ensure you embrace this new phase of your life.

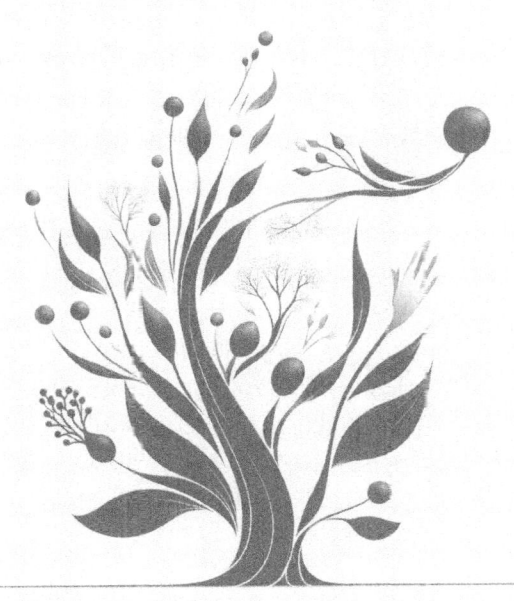

CHAPTER

Age with Elegance—Positive Aging and Proactive Health Strategies

Aging can be a difficult process to accept. Your body may feel weak and you might not be able to do the physical things you used to do easily. Your muscles have become weak and your bones are so brittle that even the slightest fall could result in fractures. You might even wake up with new aches and pains on an almost daily basis.

Your vision could become impaired, resulting in you needing glasses—not just for reading, but for everyday life. The same goes for hearing: You need to turn the volume on your TV up and may ask people to repeat themselves a few times and louder to hear them. You might even need hearing devices. Then, let's look at your physical appearance. Your hair could turn grey, and some might even fall out. You might get shorter, and your skin may resemble a shirt that's been lying in the back of your cupboard in desperate need of an iron. On the inside, your body is changing just as much, with fluctuating hormone levels bringing about your many symptoms of menopause.

All of these physical changes that you experience as you get older can have a big psychological impact on you. You may struggle to find a place in society where you can still add value—not just to your own life, but also to the lives of the people around you. This can result in feelings of frustration, anger, and even worthlessness. You might even grieve the majority of your life being over, or the loss of your life as knew it.

However, if you change the way in which you view aging and approach this new phase of your life with a positive attitude, you can find a new purpose to your life and thrive during the years to come.

Embrace Aging With a Positive Attitude

Some cultures view their elders as sources of incredible wisdom and guidance, while others see them as burdens on society. The latter likely measures value by youth or physical appearance. If you fall in this group, you might struggle even more to come to terms with the effects that aging will have on your physical, emotional, and mental health.

Unfortunately, as we've discussed, aging is inevitable, like death and taxes. While there's no cure for getting older, you can lessen the effect that this will have on you by having a healthy lifestyle (as discussed in the previous chapter) and embracing aging with a positive attitude.

Positive aging is defined as "The process of maintaining a positive attitude, feeling good about yourself, keeping fit and healthy, and engaging fully in life as you age." A recent study showed that people over the age of 50 who are satisfied with their lives have a 43% lower risk of premature death (*Positive Attitude About Aging Could Boost Health*, 2022). This is because these people have a reduced risk of serious illness, which includes cardiovascular diseases, diabetes, cancer, and stroke. Also, their cognitive abilities remained intact for much longer, lowering their chances of developing dementia and similar disorders. People who are content with their lives are also more inclined to be physically active and seek out happiness in every phase of their lives, which improves their overall mental wellness.

This shows the important connection between your mindset and your view of life with your physical and mental health.

Develop a Healthy Mindset

Renowned U.S. psychologist Carol Dweck has done extensive research on what motivates people and has come to the conclusion that people, in general, have one of two mindsets—fixed or growth (Dweck, 2016):

- **Fixed mindset:** People with a fixed mindset believe that their abilities are set in stone. If they aren't able to do something, they can't learn the necessary skills to overcome their challenges. They fear failure to such a degree that it debilitates them and keeps them from putting themselves out there to achieve success.

- **Growth mindset:** People with a growth mindset believe that they can achieve anything they put their minds to and learn all the skills necessary to reach their goals. They are dedicated to their cause and willing to put in the hard work to get there. They don't shy away from challenges and see setbacks as opportunities to learn.

Now, let's look at how these mindsets can affect your journey through menopause and aging. If you have a fixed mindset about aging, you'll believe that nothing you do can improve your ability to manage your symptoms of menopause or overcome the many challenges that aging may bring. But, if you approach this phase of your life with a growth mindset, you'll believe that not only are you capable of finding ways to reduce the impact that your symptoms of menopause and effects of aging will have on your life, but also that you can find enjoyment during this phase of life. This growth mindset will serve as a constant reminder that you can overcome whatever life might throw your way.

Tying into having a growth mindset is learning the power of the word "yet." This word has the amazing power to turn any potentially negative situation into a positive. For example, if hot flashes are one of the symptoms you struggle with the most, you might tell yourself something like, *I haven't found a way of managing my hot flashes*. But you can change this into something a lot more positive by simply adding the word "yet"—for example, *I haven't found a way of managing my hot flashes* yet. This will immediately remind you that even though you haven't been able to accomplish something in the past, it doesn't mean that you can't achieve that in the future. You are never too old to try new things you haven't done yet or learn a new skill you haven't been able to master in your past. It's all about finding the balance in your life and approaching your struggles with a positive growth mindset.

Tips for Maintaining Vitality and Resilience

While it may seem relatively easy enough to know you should approach your challenges with positivity, making this mindset change can be surprisingly difficult, especially when your struggles seem overwhelmingly big. However, if you follow these easy steps, you can overcome any challenges you might face in your life, including your journey through menopause:

- Pay close attention to yourself and what your inner critic is telling you. This will help you become more aware of your thoughts and potential limiting beliefs you might have about yourself and your life. Once you know you're allowing this negativity into your life, you can determine whether there's any evidence to back up these thoughts. If there aren't, you'll know that there isn't any truth to these unhelpful beliefs and that you shouldn't allow these to influence your life. If you do find evidence, you'll know which aspects of your life you need to work on to improve your life.

- This leads us to the second point I want to make: Always remember that you have a choice in everything you do. You can choose what influence your challenges will have on your life and which mindset approach you want to take to overcome these difficulties and challenge the way in which you view them.

- Once you've changed how you view your struggles, you can take the appropriate action to not only overcome these, but also to find happiness despite what you might be facing. Think about what actions will take you closer to your goals and what the potential implications of your actions might be. This will help you prepare for all possible outcomes and enable you to make informed decisions over what you want in your life.

- When you create plans to go for your goals, you may feel overwhelmed over the size of your goals and what you have to do to reach your desired outcome. But, if you break these goals down into smaller, easy-to-complete steps, you'll be able to reach a lot more outcomes.

- Always aim at finding and maintaining a sense of purpose that aligns with what you believe in. Knowing why you're doing something and how this fits in with your values will motivate you to give it your all and do whatever you can to reach your goals.

- When you're adopting a positive growth mindset, you also decide to dismiss any negative stereotypes you might have about aging and menopause. For example, while it's often accepted that poor physical health or strength is inevitable as you grow older, you can choose to dismiss this as a misconception and actively work on improving your physicality.

- Keep your mind active by constantly trying new activities and learning skills you haven't accomplished yet. Perhaps you want to start doing needlework or learn how to do pottery. Maybe you've always wanted to do woodwork. If you embrace these challenges and teach yourself a new skill, you'll not only empower yourself to do something you've never done before, but you'll also keep your cognitive ability strong.

- Never disregard the benefits that social interaction can bring. Many people live a life of isolation as they grow older, particularly when their children start to leave the house or when their partner dies. If you actively work on interacting with others, you'll gain a togetherness and connection with others, which will greatly benefit your mental health.

- Differentiate between what you have control over and what you can't change. There will always be times when things happen that you don't have control over. In these moments, the only thing you may be able to change is your own reaction to the event.

- Teach yourself to become more comfortable with being uncomfortable. There will always be situations in life when you are forced to step outside of your comfort zone. If you practice coping in these type of environments, you'll be able to overcome the challenges that these situations can bring a lot more effectively. Some easy ways of teaching yourself to practice mind over matter and become more comfortable with being uncomfortable include:

  - Turn the water cold toward the end of a shower. Not only will this help you understand that you can make it through a situation your body feels uncomfortable in, but ending a shower will cold water is also beneficial for your skin and closing your pores that opened by the steam of the hot water.

  - After you dish your plate of food for supper, wait around five minutes before you eat. Allow your body to truly feel the hunger pangs and reward yourself for pushing through these uncomfortable moments by enjoying your food after the five minutes have passed.

  - Turn down the heat on a very cold day or switch off the air conditioner when it's hot outside. Putting yourself in uncomfortable temperatures can help you develop the resilience you need to push through challenges you don't enjoy.

- Make sure you go for regular medical checkups so that you can treat any potential medical conditions as early as possible to prevent any of these from becoming major, life-altering concerns.

While you're working on improving your mindset and becoming more resilient to your challenges, you're likely to experience many emotional ups and downs. If having extreme mood swings is one of the symptoms of menopause you're experiencing, regulating these strong emotions can be even more difficult. In the next chapter, we'll discuss strategies you can use to improve the way in which you manage your feelings.

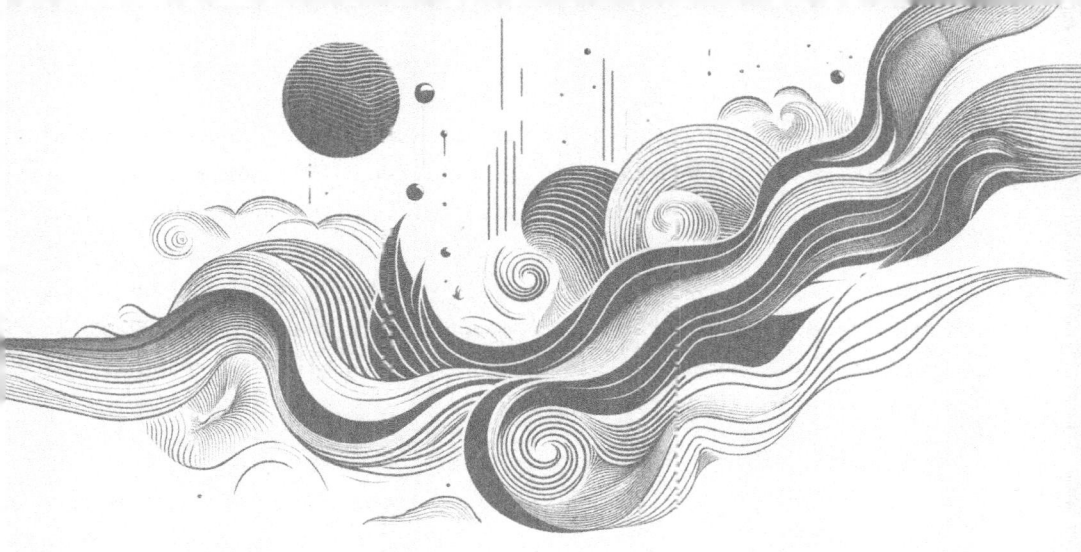

Chapter 7

Emotional Resilience—Navigating Mood Swings and Mental Health

When I say that the journey through menopause can be a massive emotional rollercoaster, I'm most certainly not exaggerating. In the same way you have no control over the movements while you're enjoying the ride at an amusement park, you have very little control over your emotions when you're going through menopause. There were many days when I went from being happy and content the one minute to being giddily excited the next, only to burst into tears for no apparent reason. It was an extremely frustrating time—not just for me but also for my family, friends, and even coworkers.

Understanding that my extreme mood swings were a result of my fluctuating hormones made it slightly easier to deal with. However, that didn't exactly stop my outbursts or the damage my emotional dysregulation was causing my relationships. I have to honestly say that overcoming my mood swings was likely my biggest challenge in menopause. Luckily, I never gave up and discovered valuable techniques that I'll share with you now and that really helped to improve my emotional regulation and mental health.

Understand Your Mood Swings

Unless you've been really lucky, you likely don't have to think very hard to remember how unpleasant your monthly premenstrual syndrome (PMS) was during your monthly cycle. Unfortunately, this can seem like nothing in comparison to the mood swings you might experience during menopause. In fact, around 4 out of 10 menopausal women experience symptoms that are more severe than PMS (Silver, 2023). Apart from the severity of these mood swings, the instability and irregularity of menopausal mood swings makes it even more difficult to deal with, as unlike PMS, these won't just flair up around the time of your cycle.

These mood swings aren't caused only by your fluctuating hormones, but also by the impact that your symptoms may have on your life and mental health. As we've said, these mood swings can also affect your relationships with the people around you, which can include your colleagues, or even your boss at work, which can have a massive influence on the progression of your career and your happiness at work.

Unfortunately, the damage that these mood swings can do to your life can cause serious mental health concerns, as you may feel isolated from others due to constantly fighting with everyone in your life. Some of the ways your mood swings can impact your mental health include:

- constant anger
- feelings of sadness
- anxiety
- depression
- forgetfulness
- difficulty concentrating
- lack of confidence
- fatigue

While your menopause could be the most obvious reason why you're having trouble managing your emotions, you should never disregard any decline in your mental health. If your struggles result in developing a serious mental illness, it's vital that you seek professional help immediately. Studies have shown that around 20% of menopausal women experience complete symptoms of depression (Begum, 2023). Always be open with your doctor about your mental health and any concerns you might have.

As we've mentioned, your family members and close friends—generally the people you're closest with—will often be on the receiving end of your mood swings. This can go two ways: The people who give you the most support may, unintentionally, be the target of your emotional onslaught or outbursts; or you could result in this over-the-top manner as a result of not receiving enough support. If you have a lot of stress in your life, as discussed in Chapter 4, you might struggle even more to keep your feelings under control.

While you're at work, you might feel like you're constantly in the spotlight. If you're experiencing brain fog as a symptom of menopause, you might lack the confidence you used to have in your work. This can be another reason why you could struggle to control yourself and your behavior while you're at work.

Trying to control your emotions by yourself can be extremely exhausting, especially when you either don't have the proper support or have specific techniques that you're following. You might end up apologizing for things that aren't your fault, avoid people you love out of fear that you'll hurt them, or live with deep regrets over your actions. All of these can impact your mental wellness even more.

Manage Your Emotions

When it comes to managing your emotions to reduce the impact that your mood swings have on your life, you can't simply try to bite your tongue, keep things bottled up, or simply hope you'll get over it without metaphorically biting someone's head off. The reality is that these emotions are even more difficult to control than ever before, especially once your mental health is affected by this. Some of the techniques that have helped me improve my emotional regulation include:

- **Keep a symptom diary.** I kept a diary on me at all times where I would record all my symptoms of menopause as well as how it affected me and what the consequences of my actions were. This helped me to not only better understand my various symptoms and behavioral patterns, but also to change how I wanted to respond to certain events and symptoms. This will also help you realize when your symptoms are getting out of hand and when you need additional help handling your struggles.

- **Dress in layers.** Keeping a symptom diary helped me realize that my hot flashes were directly linked to many of my mood swings. When I was burning up for no apparent reason, I would lash out at everyone around me. I started to always dress in layers so that I could take off clothes whenever I felt a hot flash coming on. I also invested in a battery-operated mini-fan that I kept in my handbag to cool myself off, as well as extra antiperspirant and perfume to help keep me fresh and confident.

- **Stay organized.** You may wonder how being more organized can influence your ability to manage your mood swings. It's quite simple: If you're physically organized, you free yourself from a lot of mental clutter you carry around with you. When you have fewer things to think about, you will be able to pay more attention to emotions, which can help to improve your emotional regulation. I scheduled time every week to organize and declutter my physical spaces. While it didn't necessarily show immediate results, I am convinced this helped me tremendously.

- **Talk to someone.** We all need someone we can talk to, regardless of what happens and who will understand what we're going through. A friend of mine who was going through the same stage of menopause and I decided to do weekly check-ins to make sure we were both coping with our struggles.

We would also phone each other whenever we felt like our emotions (or any other symptom of menopause) were getting the better of us. We were each other's sounding boards and would tell each other straight when we believed the other one was unreasonable or overreacting. Even though this wasn't always nice to hear, it helped us apologize to the people we hurt straight away and avoid a lot of conflict.

- **Accept your emotions.** This was another technique that was quite difficult in the beginning. When we experience big, uncomfortable emotions, it can be easy to either react to them or try to avoid them. However, if you accept your emotions, you put yourself in a position where you can stop fighting against your feelings. This can help to give you the upper hand over your feelings; you can choose how you want to respond to your accepted feelings without instinctively reacting to them in a negative way. To accept my feelings, I found it helpful to name each emotion out loud. For example, when I felt like screaming at my husband, I would hit pause and simply tell myself, *I'm feeling very angry right now*. This minute of pause and saying the name of my emotion out loud helped to remind me that what I was feeling was only an emotion and that I had the power within me to choose the outcome. Saying it out loud also helped the other person involved (in this case, my husband) understand what I was experiencing, so that the times when I failed at controlling my feelings, my outbursts didn't come as a complete shock to him.

- **Find a healthy outlet.** When we are constantly feeling strong negative emotions, having an outlet for these feelings can be extremely helpful. I used my creativity to release my built-up anger and frustration. I've never been exceptionally artistic, but I invested in a few canvasses, paint brushes, and paint, and when I felt too emotional, I would close myself in a room and just paint. Some of these paintings were so horrible that I threw them away, while others I hung proudly in my house. Ultimately, it wasn't about creating art but, rather, having an outlet for my strong feelings.

- **Learn to ride the wave.** Think of your emotions as the waves of the ocean. Take a moment to visualize how the waves build momentum and increase in size until it finally breaks. Then, the wave starts to lose momentum until it finally recedes from the shoreline. Nothing you do can stop the natural flow of the wave. Our emotions are very similar. We start calmly, with the emotion gradually building momentum, until we reach the breaking point. This is when we typically have outbursts. However, if we are able to resist the urge of lashing out at others, our emotion will lose momentum and naturally fade away. Just like a wave won't do any damage if you stay out of its way, your emotions won't hurt the people around you if you don't react to them.

Regardless of how bleak your situation may look or how strong your emotions may be, there will always be something positive you can focus on. All you need to do is choose to see the positivity in your circumstances. If you don't do this, you may find your mental health declining, which can become a serious concern.

Modern Approaches to Mental Wellness

Many people are stuck in what may be considered archaic ways of dealing with mental health problems. This can include going for therapy that might not always be as effective as you'd like it to be or pumping your body full of strong prescription medication that could have serious side effects. However, there are various modern approaches to mental wellness that you can follow to preserve your well-being and deal with any issues you may have. Let's look at seven major perspectives of modern psychology and how these can relate to helping you overcome the challenges that your menopause might bring:

- **The psychodynamic perspective:** This relates to the role that your unconscious mind, your experiences from your childhood, and your relationships with others play on how you behave in different environments. In this perspective, the mind is broken up into three key elements: the id that relates to your unconscious desires and urges; the ego that consciously deals with the challenges you face; and the superego, where your morals, values, and ideals are managed. This basically means that many of our behaviors are predetermined either by our unconscious mind or trauma from our past. If you want to work according to this perspective to overcome your challenges, you need to become more aware of your thoughts, as these could give you greater insights into your unconscious mind as well as traumatic events from your past that are still influencing your present and future. You may find that many of your emotional triggers are a result of past trauma you experienced. Identifying these triggers can go a long way in improving your emotional regulation.

- **The behavioral perspective:** This refers to the behaviors that are learned over the course of our lives that have major impacts on our lives, whether in a negative or positive manner. They are adopted either as a result of the environments we find ourselves in, peer pressure we might face, or even habits we may have. When you want to use this perspective to improve your life and your emotional regulation, you need to pay close attention to how you typically react in various situations and then compare this with the more helpful and positive ways you want to respond to these emotions. Making a conscious decision to behave in a different way to what you've learned to do will take deliberate effort and practice.

- **The cognitive perspective:** This perspective relates specifically to the mental processes that are part of your life and includes your memory, thoughts, language, decision-making, and problem-solving. It looks at how your thoughts are impacting your behavior and suggests that in order to change any of your typical reactions to things, events, or emotions, you need to first adapt your thoughts accordingly or identify any self-limiting beliefs you may have about yourself or your situation. For example, if you believe you won't be able to overcome the challenges that your menopause may bring, you'll be se stuck in your limiting beliefs about your situation and abilities that you won't be able to find working solutions to your problems or make decisions that will help push you forward.

- **The biological perspective:** This perspective has to do with how your biology—your genetics, brain, immune system, nervous system, and endocrine system—influences your behavior and your ability to reach the outcomes you desire. For example, if you have a genetic predisposition for substance abuse, you might make yourself believe that you're bound to become addicted at some point in your life, making it more difficult to resist peer pressure or any urges you have to do something. Similarly, if you come from a family that struggles with obesity, you might give up on trying to maintain a body weight, which will make dealing with the unpleasant symptoms of menopause even more difficult. Also, you may give up on improving your fluctuating hormone levels and simply decide that it's part of aging. If you do this, you'll miss out on the many benefits HRT or natural remedies can bring.

- **The cross-cultural perspective:** This perspective looks at how behaviors differ across different cultures as well as the impact that our cultural beliefs can have on our thoughts and emotions. These can have a massive influence, not only on how we view and feel about ourselves, but also on our ability to effectively deal with the challenges we face. For example, if you grow up in a strict patriarchal hierarchy, you might believe that, as a women, you should focus on your tasks while suffering in silence, or even that taking HRT may change who you are as a person. I would recommend that you discuss any cultural perspectives you have with your doctor to ensure that the decisions you make are based on scientific facts.

- **The evolutionary perspective:** This perspective relates to how different principles of evolution, such as natural selection, can affect your way of thinking as well as your behavior and emotions. It basically means that there are many parts of us, such as behavioral patterns or thought processes, that were necessary for past generations but that we no use for in the present, either due to our environments being different or simply us outgrowing these. However, if you hold onto old believes or behavioral patterns you no longer need, you'll fill your mind with unnecessary mental clutter, which can not only hamper your daily life but also affect your mental health. Again, if you're more aware of the thoughts and beliefs that consume you, you can differentiate between the ones that add value to your life and the unhelpful ones, and work on eradicating the unnecessary ones from your mind.

- **The humanistic perspective:** This final perspective looks at the role motivation plays in your thoughts, emotions, and behaviors and the influence this can have on your ability to change and achieve your desired outcomes. It's about discovering what makes you gain the personal growth necessary to change, realize your potential, and do what you can and need to in order to live by your values. It also focuses on self-acceptance, which can help you push through many of the challenges you might face. Think about what motivates you to go for your goals, whether it's to achieve a certain outcome at work, in your personal life, or your journey through menopause. What can you do to increase your motivation even more?

Understanding these seven perspectives and honing into the most applicable one when you are facing adversities can help you find the necessary solutions a lot easier. Whenever I have to overcome a challenge, I spend some time to box this difficulty into one of these perspectives before I begin to plan how I want to deal with it. This helps to direct my thinking and improve my understanding of my challenge, my ability to overcome it, and develop my game plan to reach my outcomes. After doing this for a while, boxing in your challenge will feel almost as natural as brushing your teeth every morning.

Encourage Self-Care

Women, especially mothers, are often self-sacrificial. Societal expectations make us believe that we should sacrifice our own needs to take care of others, whether it be our children, partners, friends, or aging parents. As a result, we are made to believe that practicing self-care is a selfish act, as you'll spend your time focusing on yourself rather than fulfilling the needs of others. However, as the saying goes, "You can't pour from an empty cup"—you need to take care of yourself so that you can be there for the people in your life.

Think of taking your seat in an airplane, ready for take-off. As the airline staff do their safety instructions or play the standard safety video, you'll be advised to always place the oxygen mask on yourself before you help a fellow passenger. No matter what airline your travel on, how big the plane is, or whether you sit in economy or first class, the message is always the same. In life, this oxygen mask can be a metaphor for self-care. If you don't take care of yourself first, you won't be able to take care of anyone else. Self-care is, therefore, not a selfish act, but an act of love—not just for yourself but also those around you.

Self-care is never more vital than when you go through menopause and have to undergo many changes: physically, emotionally, and mentally. If you don't focus on yourself, these changes could overwhelm you. Now, you may wonder what self-care entails. While yes, it does include finding ways to relax and seek enjoyment in life, it goes further than that. It's also about taking care of yourself mentally, physically, emotionally, socially, and spiritually. In order to care for your health and well-being, it is important to find a balance that allows you to address each of these areas. Sometimes you might need more self-care in one specific area to restore balance or find relief from a stressor in your life.

The five pillars of self-care fall into the following areas:

- **Physical:** As we discussed earlier in this book, you need to take care of your physical body so that your life can run smoothly. Always remember that there is a direct link between your body and mind: If you are in good physical health, your mental wellness will also be good. Things to consider when you're practicing physical self-care include making sure you eat well, getting enough quality sleep, doing regular exercise, going for frequent health checkups, and taking any medication that your doctor might prescribe you.

- **Social:** Being social with other people is another important aspect of self-care. When life gets busy, we often make the mistake of isolating ourselves, rushing from the one task to the next. This might result in us only spending time with work colleagues and our direct families. Unfortunately, colleagues move on to different companies and our children will eventually move out of our homes, leaving us alone, which is why it's important to make social connections outside of our workplace or homes. Having good friendships will give you a sense of belonging and connectedness as well as a support system during challenging times. Friends will be able to give you advice, be a shoulder to cry on during difficult times, and someone who can share in your joy and celebrate your successes with you.

- **Mental:** Your thoughts and the things you allow to fill your minds can have a massive impact on your emotional and mental well-being. Taking care of your mind means doing things to not only declutter mentally but also stay sharp. Activities you might consider include puzzles, learning new skills, reading a good book, or watching a movie that intrigues you or make you think, rather than simply just passing time.

- **Spiritual:** Taking care of your spiritual being doesn't mean only practicing the religion of your choice. It can also mean doing things that give your life purpose or provide you with a deeper understanding or meaning. It can include meditating, attending a religious service, or even just journaling about your life and your experiences. Ultimately, it's more about finding fulfillment than anything else.

- **Emotional:** As discussed earlier in this chapter, learning how to deal with uncomfortable or over-the-top emotions is important regardless of the phase of life you're in. However, when you're experiencing mood swings as part of menopause, emotional regulation can become more challenging than ever before. While simply acknowledging and accepting your emotions can be a form of emotional self-care, you can also add talking to a friend about your feelings, journaling, or doing leisure activities (I enjoy doing arts and crafts) to help you process and cope with your feelings.

As you can probably already deduce, practicing regular self-care holds many different benefits for your life and your health, which include:

- Reducing your stress, anxiety, and depression
- Boosting your resilience
- Increasing your happiness
- Reducing your risk of burnout
- Boosting your energy levels
- Overcoming your challenges
- Building stronger relationships with yourself and others

To ensure you gain these benefits in your life, I encourage you to develop a self-care plan tailored to your lifestyle and needs. Let's look at steps you can follow to do this:

- **Think about your needs.** Make a list of the different aspects of your life and the areas you feel you should work on most. Prioritize these different aspects or areas so that you can start working on the ones that will bring the most benefit to your life. What activities do you currently do? How can you incorporate more self-care into your daily life? How much time do you realistically have to spend on these self-care activities? Is it at all possible to create more time in your schedule for self-care?

- **Assess your stressors.** Once you've compiled your list of areas you want to work on, think about the different stressors you experience in each one that can either make self-care difficult, or keep you from gaining the maximum benefits in each. What are the true causes of your stress? Discovering the actual reason for your stress will help you to address the stressor and not just the symptom of your stress.

- **Consider self-care strategies.** Now that you know what aspects of your life you want to work on and what stressors you face in each of them, think about the strategies you can incorporate into your life to improve it. How can you fit these strategies into your schedule? There's no point in having an elaborate list of strategies if, realistically, you only have time for a few every week. The more realistic you can be in creating your list, the better your chances will be of pushing through with your strategies to gain the desired outcome.

- **Plan for difficulties.** It's inevitable that you'll face challenges on your journey to self-care, regardless of the type of activities you do or how well you schedule them. If you can plan for these challenges, you'll set yourself up for success as you'll immediately know how you want to respond to them.

- **Take small steps.** Have you ever heard the famous saying "Rome wasn't built in a day"? Neither was a proper self-care routine. No matter how motivated you may be to take better care of yourself, you need to be realistic about what you set out to achieve. Taking small steps is a good start to ensuring you're not trying to overachieve and give up before you start to experience the benefits in your life. For example, choose one aspect of your life or self-care routine that you want to focus on and make sure you do activities that not only fit into your schedule but are quick and easy to do. Over time, you can add more areas and activities to your self-care routine.

Always practice self-compassion while on your journey to self-care. On some days, you may be able to easily take care of yourself, while on other days, it will feel like a drag to just do the simplest activity. This is particularly the case on days when your symptoms of menopause peak. However, just stick to it and believe in the process. You will get there. Also, create a habit of practicing gratitude. I created a ritual in my home where every night, when we sit down for supper, each member of my family would name one thing they are grateful for. This not only helped us to become more introspective but also seek out the many good and positive things we already have.

While practicing gratitude, I was surprised at how many times my husband and I would mention each other and what we do not only for each other but also our family. Even though we've always had a great understanding and marital friendship, our intimate life did suffer as we got older and especially when my symptoms of menopause became more severe. Hearing how much we still meant to each other despite not having a roaring sex life made us both determined to work on our relationship. We found many strategies to overcome the challenges in our marriage, which we'll discuss in the next chapter.

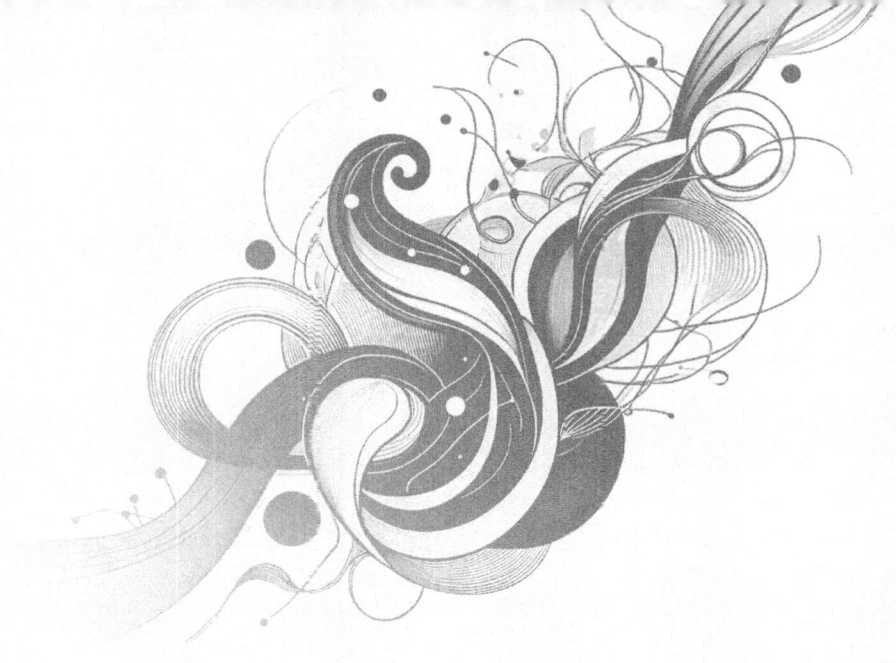

Chapter 8

Relationships Reimagined— Fostering Connection and Intimacy

During your early adult life, your sex life is likely synonymous with taking the necessary precautions not to get pregnant. Then, after you have children, you don't only have to worry about getting pregnant again but also your little ones walking in on you. Then, your monthly period can also get in the way of you having the sex life you might want. During this time, you could actually look forward to your postmenopausal life, where you don't have to worry about when you're having your period, getting pregnant, or having kids walk in and spoil the fun.

Unfortunately, postmenopausal sex might not be as stellar as you think it should be. With a declining libido, you might struggle to get in the mood. The aches and pains you experience in your body could cause you to be reluctant to take your clothes off for sex. Once you're eventually in the motion, your vaginal dryness may make sex less enjoyable than in the past. What's more, with your vaginal elasticity declining, sex could become downright painful.

While all these changes will inevitably affect your intimate life, it doesn't have to ring in the end of your sex life. You can rekindle your intimacy, revive your relationship, and enjoy a closeness with your significant other that can be stronger than it was when you were young and in love. Let's now look at the changes you can expect in your sex life as you journey through menopause. We'll also discuss tips on how to build strong relationships—not just with your romantic partner but also with your friends.

Understanding Changes in Intimacy

Many symptoms of menopause can have a severe effect on your intimate relationship with your romantic partner. As we've mentioned, these include mood swings, lack of libido, vaginal dryness, and loss of vaginal elasticity. Apart from these physical effects, the emotional strain you may be taking during menopause can also make it more difficult to get in the mood.

Due to these changes in your body, you can't expect to have the same sex life during menopause as you might have had in your 20s and 30s. While having less sex as you age is natural, it doesn't have to result in an end to your sex life. Sex can be enjoyable, no matter how old you are or how many symptoms of menopause you experience. It is, however, important that you're realistic about his phase of your life: While around half of women in their 50s are still sexually active, this percentage drops to just 27% among women in their 70s (Kraft, 2023).

You can choose to see this statistic in one of two ways. You can focus on the 73% of women in their 70s who gave up on the enjoyment that good sex can bring and resolve that once you reach a certain age or phase in your life, it will be over for you as well. Or you can choose to review this with a positive mindset: 27% of these women have found ways to work around their challenges to still enjoy intimacy with their partners. Just like these women have been able to, you can also continue to have a happy and thriving sex life.

Sex can, however, feel different when you're older. What feels good for you now won't necessarily be the same, and because it will take longer for blood to flow to your genitals when you're getting aroused, it can make it more challenging to reach an orgasm. Foreplay and other forms of physical stimulation, as well as mental engagement, can make a big difference in getting you to that desired space. Since your partner will likely continue doing what has worked for you before you started your journey through menopause, you need to explain to them how your needs have changed and what feels good for you now. Yes, you may feel uncomfortable talking about what you prefer and how you want your partner to pleasure you, but the more openly you can talk about your desires and what feels good for you, the better your sex life will be.

Apart from telling your partner what you want, you should also consider paying your vagina a little more attention. During menopause, this important body part may become dry, itchy, and painful, and intercourse can feel like torture. While replacing your estrogen levels through HRT or other natural remedies can be helpful, the following tips can also help:

- Only wear cotton underwear—this material is breathable and will allow sufficient air flow to your vagina. It also absorbs more moisture, which will help to keep you cooler and reduce any odors that might be hanging around your lady parts.
- Wash your vulva using only water or a specially formulated feminine-hygiene soap. Normal body soap, especially scented ones, can destroy the balance of bacteria in your genitals, which can increase your risk of vaginal irritation and yeast infections.

- Consider using a water-based lubricant during sex if dryness causes discomfort or pain. Vaginal moisturizers can also help to restore some of the lost moisture in your genitals.

- Discuss your sexual challenges with your doctor or gynecologist. After doing a physical examination, which will likely include a pap smear and some blood tests, they might be able to prescribe you medication that can help to boost your sexual desire.

- Look at bringing some toys into your bedroom. I'm not suggesting that you replace your partner with a vibrator, but there are many clitoral-stimulation devices that can do wonders to get your engines going enough for you to enjoy intercourse. Eros is an FDA-approved device for menopausal women.

- Consider experimenting more. This can be with your partner in the form of foreplay or trying out different positions, or by yourself by reading erotic novels or watching an erotic film. Oral sex can also be a great form of stimulation as well as it opens the levels of communication between you and your sexual partner.

- Apart from using a good lubricant, there are many other ways you can reduce the pain you might experience during intercourse. Having a warm bath before you have sex can help you relax and increase the blood flow to your genitals. You should also tell your partner as soon as any position or movement hurts you. If you try to push through the pain, you may end up with damage or bruising on your vagina, which can take a few weeks to heal.

Always remember that sex is not the only way of being intimate with your partner. Consider other forms of intimacy, such as cuddling, holding hands, having deep conversations, or simply laughing together. You can also give each other sensual massages. Over time, and as your symptoms of menopause decrease, you may recover the fire within you.

Also, even if you don't get your period anymore, it's advisable that you continue to use contraceptives for at least a year after your period stops to prevent unwanted pregnancies if you're over the age of 50, and for two years under the age of 50. As the risk of pregnancy declines, the threat of contracting a sexually transmitted infection

(STI) will still be there. Regardless of your age or the phase of life you're in, you should always take the necessary steps to safeguard yourself from these infections. If you ever suspect that you may have an STI, you should consult your doctor as soon as possible. Many of these infections can cause serious illnesses and can even be fatal.

Building Strong Relationships

Lack of intimacy is only one of many potential problems that can affect relationships. Other symptoms, such as brain fog, can also have an impact, as you may forget important events and even struggle to maintain a proper conversation. This won't just affect your romantic relationship but also your relationship with your immediate family and most important connections.

Depending on when you had children, your menopause may coincide with the time that they leave your home to settle on their own or go to college. This can put extra strain on your relationship with them and give you a new sense of freedom during which you may not know what to do with your time. This can lead to even more frustration and feelings of loneliness.

I remember how isolated I felt at times, even when my home was filled with my husband, my children, and their friends. Despite this, there were many days when I felt deeply lonely. Many days it felt as if my husband and I lived past each other, that we were too focused on tasks we had to complete rather than our personal and relational needs. I remember one night when all our children were out visiting their friends, which gave my husband and me rare alone time at home. After a few awkward minutes where we didn't really know what to say to each other, we started reminiscing about some of our favorite memories. This gave us both the motivation to work on our relationship and strengthen the bond that we share. Some of the things we decided to do together include:

- We decided to create new rituals to help ensure that we spend more time together. For us, it included starting our day sitting on our veranda enjoying a cup of coffee without feeling rushed or being interrupted by our children and cooking together on a Friday night. Think of the rituals you can introduce into your life. Perhaps you can join each other for a walk in the afternoons or take an art class together. Maybe you can add regular date nights to your schedule. I firmly believe that the type of activity you do isn't important, but rather spending time with each other, enjoying the other person's company, and connecting with your significant other, is.

- As one of our couple rituals, we decided to do weekly check-ins on a Sunday afternoon, which is typically a calm time in our home. During these check-ins, we would talk about how we are feeling and what's happening in our lives. Then, we would also mention at least three things that we appreciate about the other person. These can be things they have done over the previous week or simply just parts of their personality or nature that we love and make a difference in our life. This helped not only to make the other person feel valued but also forced us to actively seek out the positives in each other.

- Another thing we decided to do was to give each other space to do something by ourselves or with our friends, without the other person being there. This might sound counterproductive, as you'll deliberately spend time apart to build a stronger connection, but this gave us each some time for self-care to do activities we really enjoy or to work on connecting with our friends. Having this little bit of time away from each other every now and again helped us to come back feeling refreshed and appreciate the other person even more. Being more mindful of each other's personal space motivated us to want to spend more quality time together.

- Even though my husband and I have a lot in common, we have very different interests: I absolutely love reading while my husband enjoys gaming. We wanted to give each other enough time to do these things we enjoy while still spending time together. So, we added this to our schedules: I would sit and read on the couch next to my husband while he was playing his games. Even though we didn't do our activities together, we still spent time together.

- As we paid more attention to improving our relationship, my husband and I both agreed that our schedules were so full that even when we had time to spend together, we were too tired to truly enjoy it. We decided that it was time to make some serious changes. We started with both of us giving up one activity or obligation we had. I gave up my position on the school committee while my husband gave up a sports coaching gig. This freed up

- a surprisingly large amount of time that we could either spend together or simply relax with some self-care.

- We came to the agreement that we would discuss any niggles or problems in our relationship straight away and not allow these things to become major challenges in our relationship. I must be honest that, in the beginning, it felt like this caused a lot of arguments. There was a stage when I felt like we were constantly fighting about something. However, as we worked through these challenges, we got to know each other a lot better, helping us avoid and resolve similar challenges a lot quicker in the future. Always remember that your partner can't help you if you don't tell them about the challenges you face. Having this open line of communication helped us talk about a lot of other things in life, as well, which helped strengthen our bond even more.

Always make an effort to celebrate and appreciate your partner—not just when they achieve massive successes in life but also when they do small things, such as doing the dishes or making supper. Also, help them understand the effort you're putting into improving, particularly when it comes to your symptoms of menopause. If you're working on your emotional regulation and you've been able to control your mood swings, tell them what you're doing and how you believe it's working. It may be that they are so used to you being moody that they don't notice that you've had a few calm days. Cheering each other on can also make you more forgiving when your partner is having a tough time, which can go a long way in improving your mental health and reducing feelings of anxiety, depression, and stress.

Nurturing Social Support

As we've discussed in previous chapters, it's important that you find a community that you can belong to for support, guidance, and acceptance. While you may already have this with your group of friends, these friendships may have taken strain due to your moodiness and other symptoms of menopause. Luckily, it's never too late to develop connections, either with new friends or rekindling your old friendships.

Let's look at tips that can help you foster strong connections:

- Spend at least 30 minutes per week with a friend, whether this includes doing an activity with them or simply talking on the phone. This can go a long way in building connections with them. Perhaps you can phone a friend while you're commuting to work or cooking supper. This way, connecting with a friend won't take up time.

- Consider taking a class on a skill that you've always wanted to learn or on a topic you really enjoy. This will not only help to keep you mentally active but also give you the opportunity to meet new potential friends. You can even invite an old friend to take this class with you, giving you more time to build your relationship.

- Volunteer at a nonprofit organization in your community. This, again, has three purposes: It will help you to feel like you're making a contribution and make you feel like you can still make a difference, give you a purpose, and help you to meet new people. Think about the nonprofit organizations in your area and which ones you're interested in. Perhaps you want to help out at an animal shelter or a center for elderly people. If you don't know which organizations are in your area, a quick online search or on social media can help you identify different places where you can slot in to not only make a difference but also meet new people.

- Think of the old friends you might have lost contact with or go through your friends lists on your social media accounts. See if there are any people that you want to reconnect and make contact with. Start with having conversations with them on these platforms to simply just reconnect with them and build a relationship again. Then, once you're feeling more comfortable with each other and have found a common ground to use as a foundation for your relationship, consider inviting this person to do an activity with you.

- Always make sure you have proper boundaries in place. These are the invisible lines that protect you and allow you to feel safe in your connections with others. To determine what boundaries you need to set, think about your current relationships and what makes you feel uncomfortable. If anything doesn't feel right, you may want to place boundaries to ensure that you can feel safe in your relationships with others. Also, remember that when you set a boundary with someone, it's important that you explain your boundary, why you've decided to set it, and what you want to happen. For example, if a new friend is asking too many personal questions that you don't want to answer, you can simply tell them something like, "I appreciate that you're trying to get to know me by asking me these deep, personal questions, but these are topics I don't feel talking about just yet. Can we perhaps tone it down a bit and talk more in general before we jump into these deep topics?" When you approach the situation in this way, you'll help the other person understand why you're uncomfortable and tell them straight as to what you expect to happen.

- Once you're feeling comfortable with the other person, I would highly encourage you to open up about your struggles. See what you and the other person have in common and discuss any similar challenges you have with them. For example, if this friend is also going through menopause, talk about how these symptoms are affecting you. This will not only help your friends to understand what you're going through, but it will also show them that you're someone they can talk to. This can lead to an amazing support structure, where you know you're going through similar struggles, can relate to each other, and give each other advice on things that have worked for you.

- Alter your social settings where necessary. I used to love joining my friends for a glass of wine. Unfortunately, once I started my journey through menopause, any form of alcohol caused the most horrendous hot flashes, which would even continue into night sweats. It ultimately got to the point where I didn't want to join my friends anymore because I couldn't stand feeling sweaty and being embarrassed. Since get-togethers over wine was our norm, and I couldn't stand how it affected me, I became severely antisocial. Eventually, I made the mindset change where I understood that there were many other ways in which I could see my friends without consuming wine. I decided to explain to my friends why I don't want to join them for a glass of wine but that I could do a cup of coffee or a glass of juice. They completely understood, and even though some of them still chose a glass of alcohol, no one even questioned me when I ordered sparkling water instead of my normal glass of red. It's important that you do things and activities that you feel comfortable with and communicate your challenges to your friends; this will help you to be more willing to build your connection with them. Good friends will understand and want to meet you where you're happy.

- Create a rule of saying "yes" to something you're invited to that you haven't done before. Yes, this will put you out of your comfort zone, which may feel like going against the advice from the previous point, but it will also make your point of reference bigger. Perhaps you'll be invited to a new activity that you'll really enjoy, but if you weren't willing to put yourself out there, you would never have known.

- Sometimes the simplest thing you can do to build proper relationships with others is to smile. Smiling not only boosts your mood and relieves stress, but it is also contagious. When you smile at someone, whether it's someone you know or a stranger, chances are good they will smile back at you. A simple smile can be a wonderful way of creating an instant connection with others. While a simple smile won't be enough to result in a proper relationship, it can be a great starting point in going deeper.

- Think about the type of friends you want in your life and also the type of friend you'd want to be for others. What amazing qualities do you bring you to your relationships? Why do others want to be friends with you? If you can have a better understanding of the value you bring to others and why they want you to be part of their lives, you'll be able to adjust your expectations as well as how you approach your role. This can give you great confidence in your interactions with others.

Always remember that you are the master of your life. You are the only one who can determine how you approach the difficulties in your life and what steps you take to overcome these challenges, whether it's life in general or, more specifically, your symptoms of menopause. Keeping up to date on the latest research on menopause can help you make informed decisions to the betterment of your life. In the next chapter, we'll discuss the history of menopause, how it was viewed in the past, and how the understanding of this change of life has changed over the years.

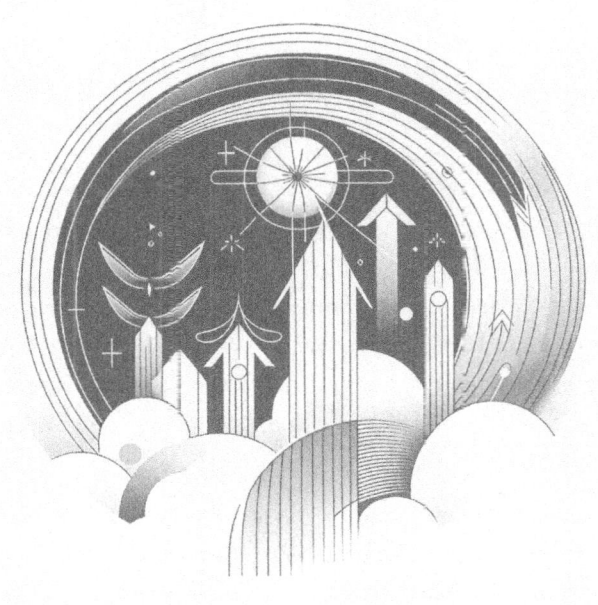

Chapter

Staying Informed and Empowered—The Future of Menopause

Chapter 9:

When you have a solid understanding of the challenges you face, you're typically able to overcome them a lot easier. Unfortunately, this is often easier said than done, particularly when it comes to a phase of life that is still being researched, such as menopause. When you look at what was understood about this phase of life a century ago and compare it to how it's viewed today, you may be shocked at the amazing strides that have already been made. If all of this development could happen over fewer than 100 years, how might the story look different in a few years?

Because of the amazing progression made, not just in the understanding of menopause, but also its treatment, I encourage you to stay up-to-date with the latest research and options available to women. I mean, if someone told me at the start of my perimenopause that I could wear a watch to control my hot flashes, I probably would've laughed in their face. Today, that is a reality for women.

In this chapter, we'll look at how the understanding of menopause has developed over the years and how it may change in the future. We'll also add a bonus section that I encourage you to ask your partner to read. Your menopause will affect your partner almost as much as it will influence your life, which is why it's not only important that they have a better understanding of what you're going through, but also that they know how they can assist you during this time.

The Evolution of Understanding Menopause

Continuous research is being done on all medical conditions, including menopause. This has a direct impact on how these conditions are viewed and treated. It's important to always stay up-to-date on the findings of this research as the way menopause is currently understood and treated may be archaic in just a few years. Specific treatments, whether it be HRT or holistic approaches, may be replaced by completely new or different forms of treatment.

Very early known documented references to menopause are scarce. This may largely boil down to a combination of menopause and its many symptoms not being understood and lifespans being shorter. Generations ago, many women might not have lived to the age of menopause or were sick with other diseases that might have other masked the symptoms of menopause, or their menopause was mistaken for other illnesses.

Centuries ago, the Greek philosopher Aristotle first observed the many changes that women go through during midlife (Singh et al., 2002). However, it was only in 1821 when the French physician Charles-Pierre-Louis de Gardanne coined the term *menopause*. Back then, the average age of menopause was believed to be 40, which was significantly younger than it is today. Even though this change of life was recognized, little was understood about the condition and its symptoms.

Just over a century later, menopause was believed to be a deficiency disease, with the major course of treatment including consuming the crushed ovaries and drinking testicular juice to replenish these deficiencies. Synthetic estrogen was also developed for the first time in 1938 but wasn't commonly used as yet. As extensive research on the topic continued over the years, it was concluded in the 1970s that this deficiency is due to declining levels of estrogen. Medical treatment for menopause was also developed, resulting in the development of HRT. The International Menopause Society was also established in the 1970s, when the first International Congress on Menopause taking place in France in 1976, with representatives from countries around the world taking part (Singh, et al., 2002).

It was then discovered that the symptoms of menopause can greatly differ depending on where you live. For example, hot flashes were regarded as one of the most common signs of menopause in Western countries, whereas it is shoulder pain in Japan and loss of vision in India. Today, the use of HRT is much more common among women in Western countries, where those in the east prefer to take natural or holistic approaches to find relief.

The Future of Menopause

While it's impossible to know what the future of menopause will look like and how it will be different from how it's viewed and treated currently, research is continuously done on the topic, making it worthwhile to stay informed to make empowered decisions about your treatment of choice. Many apps are already available to download on your phone to track your symptoms of menopause, which helps you to stay in control of your health, symptoms, and treatment.

As the understanding of menopause increases, so is the empathy of greater society toward women who go through this change in life. While many women were historically told to just "deal with it" when they struggled with symptoms of menopause, this is no longer the case, as the understanding of menopause has greatly improved.

While it's always best to have your menopause diagnosed by a physician, who will most likely do a variety of tests and examinations to confirm this change in life, there are many online quizzes available where you can test the likelihood that you've entered this phase of life. You can even purchase watch-like devices that cool the skin on the inside of the wearer's wrist, lowering their body temperature and reducing the impact that hot flashes can have. Whether this really works or not, I can't guarantee, but a friend of mine invested in one of these and she absolutely swears by it.

Whether any other breakthroughs will come in the form of menopause relief remains to be seen. At the time of publication, there were groups advocating for up to 20 days' paid leave per year for women going through menopause to use on days when their symptoms are severe. Only time will tell if these groups' attempts at liberating women will be successful.

Menopause From the Male Perspective

Menopause can be a challenging time for everyone involved, especially the partner of the woman on this journey. Unfortunately, many of these spouses simply don't understand what their wives are going through and may even believe that their wives should simply "get over it." I remember how frustrated my husband used to get with me, both when my symptoms were getting the better of me and when my menopause affected him and our sex life. If you have a partner that is similarly annoyed by your change in life, this last section is for them. For the purpose of this book, we'll refer to your partner as male, but if you have a female life partner who hasn't gone through menopause yet, they will also find value out of learning more about this phase of life.

Gentlemen, you may have heard people use the word "menopause" with the similar level of disgust many regard swear words. While some view this change in life in that way, understanding what your partner is going through will help you to be more sympathetic toward her struggles. Instead of getting annoyed by her tossing and turning at night due to insomnia or night sweats, you'll understand that she can't help it, and perhaps you'll even be more willing to add an extra blanket when she insists on having the air conditioner or fan on in the middle of winter.

In a nutshell, menopause happens when your partner experiences drastic hormonal changes (estrogen and progesterone), which signals the end of her productive life. While the end of her menstrual cycle is typically a sure sign that she has reached menopause, this change of life can start years before that with symptoms that can include:

- hot flashes
- night sweats
- fatigue
- difficulty sleeping
- decreased sex drive
- vaginal dryness
- mood swings
- decreased concentration
- memory lapses or brain fog

Most women will start with these symptoms in their 40s, although it isn't unusual for women to start perimenopause, the first stage, in their 30s. Others might only show the first signs well into their 50s. If you're married, you likely promised to be there for you wife in sickness and in health; menopause can put this promise to the test. So, let's look at specific things you can do to make this journey through this change in life easier for both of you:

- **Understand the symptoms.** While we have listed the most common symptoms above, there may be many others affecting your partner. I would highly recommend that you do a quick online search when your partner suddenly presents with a new symptom to determine whether it could be related to her menopause or a sign of something more serious. Doing this search can help you to adjust your response to her symptoms and help you prepare for what to expect.

- **Ask questions.** If you ever feel unsure about what your partner is experiencing or why she might be behaving in specific ways, ask her about it rather than simply wondering and jumping to your own conclusions. Asking questions won't just educate you on what she is going through, but it will also show her that you care and want to understand. Having these conversations about menopause can also do wonders to foster a strong connection with her. Having more insight into her symptoms could even help you come up with potential solutions or ways to minimize the impact that these have on her. It will also help you to be more empathetic to what she is going through.

- **Tread carefully.** Due to her hormonal fluctuations, your partner may struggle with severe mood swings. She may be loving and kind one minute and lashing out over the smallest things the very next. While your irritability with the situation may easily match hers, you need to try your best to stay patient with her and remember that the struggles she is going through are only temporary. If you see she is being moody or even unreasonable, give her the space she needs. Remember, she isn't being moody on purpose—it's her fluctuating hormones talking. Biting on your tongue will go a long way toward preserving the peace and your relationship.

- **Understand that sleep may be difficult.** I haven't met many people who don't enjoy having a good night's sleep or who want to struggle night after night to get some rest. Unfortunately, sleep can be challenging for women in menopause. Not only may she struggle to fall asleep, but she might also have difficulty staying asleep. Furthermore, her night sweats make sleeping uncomfortable, as well. Help her by ensuring a cool, calm environment in your room, put some ice in her water for her night, consider using sleep sounds to help her settle into good sleep, and encourage her to avoid caffeine, particularly during the afternoons and evenings. Even if she wakes you up in the night when she struggles relax, try your best not to show your frustration.

- **Never mention her weight.** Many menopausal women struggle with managing their weight and even gain a few extra pounds during these years.

This is a result of her metabolism slowing down due to the change in her hormones. Whatever you do, never mention any weight she might have gained or her struggles to lose the unwanted pounds. Instead, encourage her to follow a healthy diet, which include a proper eating plan and workout program.

- **Make time for your partner.** If you and your partner have been together for a long time, you might have to work on rekindling the spark in your relationship. Make time to spend with her by planning special date nights or simply enjoying each other's company at home. Always remind her of what she means to you, why you love her, and how beautiful she still is, even if her body looks different than it did when you started dating.

- **Roll with the punches.** Your sex life may be vastly different from what you're used to or how you'd like it to be. Instead of putting pressure on your partner to be intimate, understand that her symptoms of menopause can cause vaginal dryness, loss of elasticity, and a lack of libido. She might struggle to get into the mood, have pain during intercourse, and struggle to climax. If you're patient with her, your chances of regaining the desired level of intimacy will greatly increase rather than if you put pressure on her. Find other ways of being intimate, which can include foreplay, oral sex, or even just a good cuddle or massage without expecting a happy ending.

- **Consider the options.** There are many medications and herbal remedies that can help your partner cope with her symptoms of menopause. However, deciding which treatment to choose can be a very difficult decision to make. Help her through this process by looking at the pros and cons of all the different treatment options and, if it will help her, accompany her to the doctor to discuss her options. However, never pressure her to start a treatment program that she doesn't feel comfortable with.

Always remember that your partner is going through an extremely emotional time. These changes ring in the end of her reproductive era and the start of her midlife. She may feel upset about this and have more questions than answers. However, if you're willing to take this one day at a time and treat her with the patience and empathy she deserves, your bond can grow even stronger during this time.

Chapter 10

Your Menopause, Your Power—A Journey of Transformation

A women's body is extremely complex but probably the most amazing thing you'll find in this world. Every month, we bleed for 5–7 days, without ever bleeding out. We are able to create new life inside of our bodies, and once we give birth, our bodies create the precise nutrition our little ones need. How can anyone disagree that the female body is absolutely glorious?

Unfortunately, having this remarkable, life-giving vessel comes with a price: It's inevitable that all women will go through the various stages of menopause. Once you reach this change in life, your mindset will play a major role in how you experience the various symptoms, many of which can be rather unpleasant. You can allow your hot flashes, night sweats, severe mood swings, and vaginal dryness (to name a few) to get the better of you, or you choose to embrace this odyssey with grace and see your symptoms of menopause as a celebration of your womanhood.

Having a deep understanding of menopause, its various stages, and how the symptoms can affect you will help you prepare for what lies ahead on your journey. This knowledge will be vital when you need to decide on the best treatment options. While your doctor will advise you on what they believe will benefit you the most—be it HRT, natural remedies, or lifestyle changes—the decision will ultimately be yours. The in-depth knowledge we've discussed in this book, coupled with stories of shared experiences of other women going through the same struggles on their journeys, will empower you and give you the confidence you need to make these important decisions.

While I've shared some insights into my journey as well as stories of remarkable women I've met along the way, don't underestimate the strength you can find in your own community of women. Knowing that you're not alone, listening to what others have experienced, and sharing advice on how you can deal with having your third angry outburst within an hour of waking up will give you a sense of support and togetherness that can help you thrive throughout even the harshest of symptoms.

Always remember that you're in charge of your life, your health, and your happiness. You have blossomed through many other stages of big hormonal changes in your body, such as puberty and pregnancy. And you can do it again through menopause. I have the utmost faith in you!

Let's make *The Menopause Odyssey: From Hot Flashes to Hormonal Harmony* a call to arms, a declaration that the journey through menopause is not a solitary trek but a shared voyage, rich in challenges, triumphs, and transformative moments. Embrace the odyssey with me to navigate these waves of change with grace, empowerment, and a renewed sense of vitality.

Tools for Implementation

Having the deeper understanding of menopause and its various symptoms will enable you to not only cope with this change in life more effectively but even find enjoyment. I believe a key to achieving this is being completely aware of what's happening in your body. To help you gain this high level of awareness, we'll now look at various tools you can use in your daily life, such as a symptom tracker, a checklist for symptoms and questions for when you visit the doctor, and apps you may want to download onto your phone or tablet to ensure an effortless journey through menopause.

Perimenopause Symptom Tracker

When you start to suspect that you're starting on your journey through menopause, it can be helpful to track the various symptoms you might have. This will help you to know when you may need to go to the doctor or which symptoms you might want to consider taking treatment for. To help you with this, let's look at a perimenopause symptom tracker you can use:

Symptom	Date of first symptom	Intensity of symptom (rate it from 1 to 5)	How I tried to treat this symptom	Did it work?	What else can I try?

Symptom	Date of first symptom	Intensity of symptom (rate it from 1 to 5)	How I tried to treat this symptom	Did it work?	What else can I try?

If you ever feel unsure about whether what you're experiencing is a symptom of menopause or perhaps something completely unrelated that might need urgent attention and treatment, answering the following questions might help:

Question	Never	Often	Always
My periods are irregular.			
I struggle with PMS symptoms (bloating, cramps, headaches, breast tenderness, and irritability).			

Question	Never	Often	Always
I have difficulty falling asleep at night.			
I often wake up during the night.			
I struggle with night sweats.			
I find it difficult to regulate my emotions and control my mood swings.			
I often feel weak and tired.			
My anxiety levels are through the roof.			
I forget a lot of things.			
I struggle to concentrate on the tasks I'm busy with.			
I have digestive problems (heartburn, nausea, diarrhea, bloating, or constipation).			
I struggle with painful joints.			
I gain weight quickly despite watching what I eat.			
I struggle to lose weight.			
My libido is very low.			
I struggle with vaginal dryness.			
My hair is falling out.			
Am I treated for other medical conditions?			
I suffer fractures easily when I fall or bump into things.			
I have struggled with hormonal imbalances in the past (thyroid problems, diabetes, insulin resistance, or polycystic ovarian syndrome).			

Preparing for Your Doctor's Visit

Once you've decided that you should consult your doctor, it's best that you go well-prepared. You may feel very overwhelmed during the visit, so having a list of your symptoms and questions you want to ask them can help you gain the most value from your appointment and ensure you talk about all the potential treatment options. The table below can help you with discussing your symptoms:

Symptom	Severity of symptom	Date of first symptom	Additional information (include what you've tried, how effective it was, or how urgently you may need intervention)
Irregular menstrual cycle			
Hot flashes			
Difficulty sleeping			
Night sweats			
Elevated heart rate			
Vaginal dryness			
Discomfort during intercourse			
Low sex drive			
Urinary problems			
Mood changes			
Mental health problems			
Memory problems			
Lack of concentration			
Weight gain			
Hair loss			
Skin changes			
Other symptoms			

Next, let's look at questions you might want to ask the doctor:

- Does your practice treat menopausal women? If not, can you recommend a physician who specializes in this?

- How can I differentiate between my symptoms of menopause or those that might indicate another health concern?
- How far along am I in my journey through menopause?
- How long will my symptoms likely last?
- How will my menopause impact my overall well-being?
- Should I continue using birth control? For how long?
- What treatment can I consider using for my menopause? Which type of treatment will be best for me?
- What are the major side effects of HRT? If I opt for using HRT, how can I minimize the impact that this can have on my life?
- What influence will menopause have on my sex life?
- What can I do to make sex more enjoyable?
- What impact will my menopause have on other health conditions I have?
- Will menopause increase my risk of contracting or developing another disease or health condition? What tests or screenings can I do to either minimize my risk or pick up on a health concern early?
- What natural remedies can I use? What are the potential concerns I should be aware of when using these remedies?
- Should I make any changes to my diet? What foods should I absolutely avoid? What are the best foods to eat?
- What exercises should I do? How often should I work out?
- What lifestyle changes should I consider making to improve my life and reduce the impact that my menopause may have on my life?
- How will I know when I've reached postmenopause?

While these questions are a good starting point of what you might want answered, there are many other things you might wonder about. Add these to your personalized list of answers you're seeking and never feel bad about how many questions you ask your doctor. They are not only trained in treating these conditions, but they also understand that these change in life may be a very scary time for you.

Applications to Consider Using

There are many apps you can download to your phone or tablet on which you can track your symptoms of menopause and gain access to the latest news, research, and treatment options. Some of these can make your life a lot easier, particularly if you have brain fog and struggle to remember how your symptoms are affecting you or which tasks you need to complete.

Unfortunately, not all of these apps are made equal. Some are sponsored by specific pharmaceutical companies to promote their medication or only provide information based on a specific agenda they choose to advance. Also, some may not keep your data safe, which is something you should look into before downloading the app and entering your personal information. I always recommend people to do proper research and not simply choose the first app that pops up. If you're part of a community of menopausal women, you can also ask them about which apps they prefer using.

While there are new ones being developed all the time, a list of apps you can consider looking at include:

- **Evernow:** This app was developed according to the guidelines of the American College of Gynecology and North American Menopause Society. On this app, you'll have access to a clinician and apparently all board-certified doctors and nurses, who can suggest various symptom relief based on your individual circumstances and needs. This app promises not to disclose or sell the information of its users.

- **Midday:** This app provides complete menopause treatment and management, including symptom tracking. You can also connect this app to your Fitbit or smart watch to track your sleeping patterns and physical activity, which can give you a good overview of your overall wellness and can help you to take a more holistic approach to your treatment. For example, you'll be able to track your hot flashes, which can help you identify and avoid your various triggers. This app also gives you access to a healthcare professional in the form of virtual visits, where you not only get medical advice but also prescriptions for HRT.

- **Caria:** This is another user-friendly app that easily manages and tracks your symptoms of menopause, as well as other behavioral options, including cognitive behavioral therapy, mindful meditation, fitness trainers, life coaches, and dietitians to help you improve your overall health and help you cope with your symptoms more effectively. Experts also provide advice and insights into menopause in the form of video sessions.

- **Balance:** This app was developed in the United Kingdom by a leading menopause expert in this country, Dr. Louise Newson. As with other apps, you can track your symptoms of menopause, connect with other women, and find the support you need while on this journey.

- **Perry:** This app provides valuable insights into menopause by first asking you to complete a quiz to determine exactly where you are on your journey to menopause. After this, you'll gain access to information that is specific to your phase of life, which includes guidance by experts—fitness specialists, nutritionists, psychologists, and gynecologists. They not only focus on the physical aspects of menopause but also on mental health and taking care of your psychological wellness. This app also provides access to a marketplace, where you can order various products that are directly aimed at providing relief for many different symptoms of menopause.

Always remember that, even though these apps can provide incredible insights into menopause and coping with the various symptoms you may have, it should never replace your gynecologist or treating physician. It's still advisable that you see your doctor at least once a year for a thorough checkup and to ensure there are no other health concerns that need treating.

Glossary

- **Anti-inflammatory foods:** Specific foods that reduce the inflammation in your body. Examples include berries, avocados, nuts, fatty fish, leafy greens, peppers, and olive oil.
- **Atrophy:** The degeneration of bodily cells that typically comes with aging.
- **Estrogen:** A hormone that plays a vital role in the sexual and reproductive health of women. When the levels of this hormone start to decline, it typically signals the start of menopause.
- **Fixed mindset:** Believing that you have all the skills and ability you'll ever have and can't learn or develop new skills in your life.
- **Galveston diet:** An anti-inflammatory eating plan specifically designed for menopausal women to help them not only lose weight but also improve their overall physical wellness.
- **Growth mindset:** Believing that you can develop various skills to become the absolute best version of yourself without allowing anything to hold you back.
- **Hormonal imbalance:** Hormonal imbalance happens when there are either too many or too few specific hormones present in your body, which can result in a variety of symptoms and health conditions.
- **Hormone replacement therapy (HRT):** Medication comprising of synthetic hormones, such as estrogen and progesterone, that is used by menopausal women to reduce the severity and impact of their symptoms.
- **Hot flashes:** One of the most common symptoms of menopause, a sudden and unexpected feeling of extreme warmth, typically felt in the neck, chest, and face. It can cause redness on the skin and sweating.
- **Macronutrients:** The main sources of nutritional foods we eat, which include proteins, fats, and carbohydrates.

- **Menopause:** The change of life in a women's life that signals the end of her reproductive years. It is typically associated with the end of a woman's monthly menstrual cycle and can bring a host of different and unpleasant symptoms.
- **Micronutrients:** Food sources that are rich in vitamins and minerals and are typically consumed in small amounts.
- **Natural remedies:** Using natural sources, such as herbs and plants, for medicinal purposes to treat various conditions.
- **Ovaries:** The female reproductive organ that releases eggs for fertilization and produces hormones, such as estrogen and progesterone.
- **Ovarian failure:** When your ovaries stop functioning as they used to, which results in not releasing eggs for fertilization and low levels of female hormones, such as estrogen and progesterone.
- **Progesterone:** A female hormone that prepares the lining of the uterus for the implantation of a fertilized egg.
- **Testosterone:** Predominantly male hormone that supports libido and sexual function in women.
- **Vaginal atrophy:** A natural symptom of menopause that results in the thinning and drying of the vagina due to low levels of estrogen. It can also cause a loss of elasticity in the vagina, which often results in uncomfortable and painful sexual intercourse.

Acknowledgments:
A Note of Gratitude

Dear readers, experts, and my fellow menopausal women—

From the bottom of my heart, I would like to extend my deepest gratitude for the impact you've made in my life, either through reading my work, doing your relentless research on menopause, or simply fighting the good fight during this change in life with me. Knowing that I'm sharing this amazing journey with every one of you provides me with absolute vigor to overcome any challenges I might face.

I have found amazing strength in our communal experiences, and I hope reading about what has worked for others will also inspire and motivate you on your journey through menopause. This odyssey is anything but a solitary trek. We are all in this together, helping one another through tough times, fixing one another's crowns when necessary, and celebrating our amazing successes together.

If you found value in the content of this book, I kindly ask that you share your thoughts and reviews on Amazon so that I can not only reach more women but also expand our community of warrior women even more.

With gratitude,
Valerie

References

About hormone replacement therapy (HRT). (2023, July 21). NHS. https://www.nhs.uk/medicines/hormone-replacement-therapy-hrt/about-hormone-replacement-therapy-hrt/

Ames, H. (2022, February 22). *Natural remedies for menopause*. Medical News Today. https://www.medicalnewstoday.com/articles/natural-remedies-for-menopause

Astorino, D. (2023, May 21). *5 common menopause myths, debunked*. One Medical. https://www.onemedical.com/blog/healthy-living/5-common-menopause-myths-debunked/

Begum, J. (2023, April 7). *The emotional roller coaster of menopause*. WebMD. https://www.webmd.com/menopause/emotional-roller-coaster

Breeding, B. (2018, July 23). *Positive aging: Changing your mindset about growing older*. MyLifeSite. https://mylifesite.net/blog/post/positive-aging-changing-mindset-growing-older/

Changes in hormone levels, sexual side effects of menopause. (2019). The North American Menopause Society. https://www.menopause.org/for-women/sexual-health-menopause-online/changes-at-midlife/changes-in-hormone-levels

Christian, E. (2021, July 13). *5 tips for nurturing friendships during menopause*. Rest Less. https://restless.co.uk/health/healthy-body/5-tips-for-nurturing-friendships-during-menopause/

Cohen, M. (2022, July 26). *7 exercises you need to try if you're menopausal.* Good Housekeeping. https://www.goodhousekeeping.com/health/fitness/g40476189/menopause-exercises/

Dweck, C. (2016, January 13). *What having a "growth mindset" actually means.* Harvard Business Review. https://hbr.org/2016/01/what-having-a-growth-mindset-actually-means

Ferris, E. (2023, April 3). *Preparing for menopause: Understanding the signs and symptoms in all three stages.* Summa Health. https://www.summahealth.org/flourish/entries/2023/04/preparing-for-menopause-understanding-the-signs-and-symptoms-in-all-three-stages

Groves, M. (2018, November 23). *Menopause diet: How what you eat affects your symptoms.* Healthline. https://www.healthline.com/nutrition/menopause-diet#bottom-line

Hailes, J. (2024, January 19). *Menopause and natural remedies.* Jean Hailes for Women's Health. https://www.jeanhailes.org.au/donations

Haskey, J. (2023, April 4). *Menopause and stress.* The Menopause Charity. https://www.themenopausecharity.org/2023/04/04/menopause-and-stress/

Hormone therapy for menopause: Types, benefits & risks. (2021, June 28). Cleveland Clinic. https://my.clevelandclinic.org/health/treatments/15245-hormone-therapy-for-menopause-symptoms

Introduction to menopause. (2023, November 29). Johns Hopkins Medicine. https://www.hopkinsmedicine.org/health/conditions-and-diseases/introduction-to-menopause

Johnson, S. (2019, June 5). *How to lose weight during menopause: 10 ways.* Medical News Today. https://www.medicalnewstoday.com/articles/325386#increasing-activity

Johnson, T. C. (2022, August 11). *Menopause and good nutrition*. WebMD. https://www.webmd.com/menopause/staying-healthy-through-good-nuitrition

Kraft, C. (2023, October 30). *How sex changes after menopause*. Johns Hopkins Medicine. https://www.hopkinsmedicine.org/health/wellness-and-prevention/how-sex-changes-after-menopause

Miller, K. D. (2019, March 8). *Positive aging: 10+ principles to shift beliefs around age*. Positive Psychology. https://positivepsychology.com/positive-aging/

Nikam, S. (2021, May 18). *Galveston diet review: Rules, meal plan, and foods list*. Healthline. https://www.healthline.com/nutrition/galveston-diet

Positive attitude about aging could boost health. (2022, August 24). Harvard T.H. Chan. https://www.hsph.harvard.edu/news/hsph-in-the-news/positive-attitude-about-aging-could-boost-health/

Postmenopause: Signs, symptoms & what to expect. (2021, October 5). Cleveland Clinic. https://my.clevelandclinic.org/health/diseases/21837-postmenopause#diagnosis-and-tests

Princing, M. (2023, May 22). *Yes, menopause impacts mental health. Here's why*. Right as Rain by UW Medicine. https://rightasrain.uwmedicine.org/mind/mental-health/menopause-mental-health

Scott, E. (2023, February 12). *5 self-care practices for every area of your life*. Verywell Mind. https://www.verywellmind.com/self-care-strategies-overall-stress-reduction-3144729

Sexual wellbeing, intimacy and menopause. (2023, March 14). NHS Inform. https://www.nhsinform.scot/healthy-living/womens-health/later-years-around-50-years-and-over/menopause-and-post-menopause-health/sexual-wellbeing-intimacy-and-menopause/

Silver, N. E. (2023, April). *Mood changes during perimenopause are real. Here's what to know.* ACOG. https://www.acog.org/womens-health/experts-and-stories/the-latest/mood-changes-during-perimenopause-are-real-heres-what-to-know

Singh, A., Kaur, S., & Walia, I. (2002). A historical perspective on menopause and menopausal age. *Bulletin of the Indian Institute of History of Medicine (Hyderabad), 32*(2), 121–135. https://pubmed.ncbi.nlm.nih.gov/15981376/

Spelman, B. (2022, January 8). *The 7 perspectives in modern psychology.* Private Therapy Clinic. https://theprivatetherapyclinic.co.uk/blog/the-7-perspectives-in-modern-psychology/

Printed in Great Britain
by Amazon